Transfusion Medicine

Editors

ERIC A. GEHRIE
EDWARD L. SNYDER

HEMATOLOGY/ONCOLOGY CLINICS OF NORTH AMERICA

www.hemonc.theclinics.com

Consulting Editors
GEORGE P. CANELLOS
H. FRANKLIN BUNN

October 2019 • Volume 33 • Number 5

ELSEVIER

1600 John F. Kennedy Boulevard ● Suite 1800 ● Philadelphia, Pennsylvania, 19103-2899

http://www.theclinics.com

HEMATOLOGY/ONCOLOGY CLINICS OF NORTH AMERICA Volume 33, Number 5
October 2019 ISSN 0889-8588, ISBN 13: 978-0-323-70906-4

Editor: Stacy Eastman
Developmental Editor: Kristen Helm

Hematology/Oncology Clinics (ISSN 0889-8588) is published bimonthly by Elsevier Inc., 360 Park Avenue South, New York, NY 10010-1710. Months of issue are February, April, June, August, October, and December. Business and Editorial Offices: 1600 John F. Kennedy Blvd., Ste. 1800, Philadelphia, PA 19103–2899. Customer Service Office: 3251 Riverport Lane, Maryland Heights, MO 63043. Periodicals postage paid at New York, NY and at additional mailing offices. Subscription prices are $430.00 per year (domestic individuals), $830.00 per year (domestic institutions), $100.00 per year (domestic students/residents), $480.00 per year (Canadian individuals), $1028.00 per year (Canadian institutions) $547.00 per year (international individuals), $1028.00 per year (international institutions), and $255.00 per year (international and Canadian students/residents). International air speed delivery is included in all *Clinics* subscription prices. All prices are subject to change without notice. **POSTMASTER:** Send address changes to *Hematology/Oncology Clinics of North America*, Elsevier Health Sciences Division, Subscription Customer Service, 3251 Riverport Lane, Maryland Heights, MO 63043. Customer Service (orders, claims, online, change of address): Elsevier Health Sciences Division, Subscription **Customer Service, 3251 Riverport Lane, Maryland Heights, MO 63043. Tel: 1-800-654-2452 (U.S. and Canada); 314-447-8871 (outside U.S. and Canada). Fax: 314-447-8029. E-mail: journalscustomerservice-usa@elsevier.com (for print support); journalsonlinesupport-usa@elsevier.com (for online support).**

Reprints. For copies of 100 or more, of articles in this publication, please contact the Commercial Reprints Department, Elsevier Inc., 360 Park Avenue South, New York, New York 10010-1710; Tel.: 212-633-3874, Fax: 212-633-3820, E-mail: reprints@elsevier.com.

Hematology/Oncology Clinics of North America is covered in *MEDLINE/PubMed (Index Medicus), EMBASE/ Excerpta Medica, and BIOSIS.*

Contributors

CONSULTING EDITORS

GEORGE P. CANELLOS, MD
William Rosenberg Professor of Medicine, Department of Medical Oncology, Dana-Farber Cancer Institute, Boston, Massachusetts, USA

H. FRANKLIN BUNN, MD
Professor of Medicine, Division of Hematology, Brigham and Women's Hospital, Harvard Medical School, Boston, Massachusetts, USA

EDITORS

ERIC A. GEHRIE, MD
Assistant Professor, Pathology and Surgery, Medical Director, Blood Bank, Co-Director, Patient Blood Management Program, Associate Director, Pathology Residency Program, The Johns Hopkins Medical Institutions, Department of Pathology, Division of Transfusion Medicine, Johns Hopkins University School of Medicine, Baltimore, Maryland, USA

EDWARD L. SNYDER, MD, FACP
Professor, Laboratory Medicine, Yale School of Medicine, Director, Transfusion Medicine Services, Yale New Haven Hospital, New Haven, Connecticut, USA

AUTHORS

J. WADE ATKINS, MS, MT(ASCP) SBB, CQA(ASQ)
Supervisor, Quality Assurance and Regulatory Affairs, Department of Transfusion Medicine, Clinical Center, National Institutes of Health, Bethesda, Maryland, USA

ANDREW P. CAP, MD, PhD
Coagulation and Blood Research, U.S. Army Institute of Surgical Research, Texas, USA

SHRUTI CHATURVEDI, MBBS, MS
Assistant Professor, Division of Hematology, Department of Medicine, The Johns Hopkins Medical Institutions, The Johns Hopkins Hospital, Baltimore, Maryland, USA

KATHRYN E. DANE, PharmD
Clinical Pharmacy Specialist, Department of Pharmacy, The Johns Hopkins Hospital, Baltimore, Maryland, USA

STEVEN M. FRANK, MD
Professor, Department of Anesthesiology/Critical Care Medicine, Medical Director, Center for Bloodless Medicine and Surgery, Medical Director, Johns Hopkins Health System Blood Management Clinical Community, Faculty, The Armstrong Institute for Patient Safety and Quality, The Johns Hopkins Medical Institutions, Baltimore, Maryland, USA

ERIC A. GEHRIE, MD
Assistant Professor, Pathology and Surgery, Medical Director, Blood Bank, Co-Director, Patient Blood Management Program, Associate Director, Pathology Residency Program, The Johns Hopkins Medical Institutions, Department of Pathology, Division of Transfusion Medicine, Johns Hopkins University School of Medicine, Baltimore, Maryland, USA

RUCHIKA GOEL, MD, MPH
Adjunct Assistant Professor, Division of Transfusion Medicine, Department of Pathology, The Johns Hopkins Medical Institutions, Baltimore, Maryland, USA; Assistant Professor of Internal Medicine and Pediatrics, Division of Hematology/Oncology, Simmons Cancer Institute at SIU School of Medicine, Associate Medical Director, Mississippi Valley Regional Blood Center, Springfield, Illinois, USA

STEVEN HIGHFILL, PhD
Center for Cellular Engineering, Department of Transfusion Medicine, Clinical Center, National Institutes of Health, Bethesda, Maryland, USA

RONALD JACKUPS Jr, MD, PhD
Departments of Pathology and Immunology, Washington University School of Medicine, St Louis, Missouri, USA

OLIVER KARAM, MD, PhD
Division of Pediatric Critical Care Medicine, Department of Pediatrics, Children's Hospital of Richmond at VCU, Richmond, Virginia, USA

KIMBERLY A. KASOW, DO
Associate Director for the UNC Bone Marrow Transplant and Cellular Therapy Program Quality Initiatives, Department of Pediatrics, The University of North Carolina at Chapel Hill, Chapel Hill, North Carolina, USA

DAVID A. LEIBY, PhD
Chief Product Review Branch, Division of Emerging and Transfusion Transmitted Diseases, FDA/CBER/OBRR, Silver Spring, Maryland, USA

JOHN LINDSLEY, PharmD
Clinical Pharmacy Specialist, Department of Pharmacy, The Johns Hopkins Hospital, Baltimore, Maryland, USA

ZHEN MEI, MD
Pathology Resident, University of Chicago Medicine, Chicago, Illinois, USA

MANUELA PLAZAS MONTANA
Research Program Assistant, Division of Hematology, Department of Medicine, Johns Hopkins University School of Medicine, Baltimore, Maryland, USA

MARIANNE E. NELLIS, MD, MS
Division of Pediatric Critical Care Medicine, Department of Pediatrics, NewYork-Presbyterian Hospital - Weill Cornell Medicine, New York, New York, USA

SANDHYA R. PANCH, MD
Center for Cellular Engineering, Department of Transfusion Medicine, Clinical Center, National Institutes of Health, Bethesda, Maryland, USA

KRISTIN M. REDDOCH-CARDENAS, PhD
Coagulation and Blood Research, U.S. Army Institute of Surgical Research, San Antonio, Texas, USA

OPAL REDDY, MD
Center for Cellular Engineering, Department of Transfusion Medicine, Clinical Center, National Institutes of Health, Bethesda, Maryland, USA

LINDA M.S. RESAR, MD
Professor, Department of Medicine (Hematology), Oncology and Institute for Cellular Engineering, The Johns Hopkins Medical Institutions, Co-Director, Center for Bloodless Medicine and Surgery, Baltimore, Maryland, USA

JOHN D. ROBACK, MD, PhD
Professor and Vice-Chair for Clinical Pathology, Department of Pathology and Laboratory Medicine, Emory University School of Medicine, Atlanta, Georgia, USA

NAREG H. ROUBINIAN, MD, MPHTM
Division of Research, Kaiser Permanente Northern California, Oakland, California, USA; Vitalant Research Institute, University of California, San Francisco, San Francisco, California, USA

SARA J. RUTTER, MD
Department of Laboratory Medicine, Yale University School of Medicine, New Haven, Connecticut, USA

THOMAS G. SCORER, MBBS, FRCPath
School of Cellular and Molecular Medicine, University of Bristol, Bristol Royal Infirmary, Bristol, United Kingdom; Centre of Defence Pathology, Royal Centre for Defence Medicine, Birmingham, United Kingdom

SATISH SHANBHAG, MBBS, MPH, FACP
Associate Professor of Medicine and Oncology, Division of Hematology, Department of Medicine, Johns Hopkins University School of Medicine, Baltimore, Maryland, USA

EDWARD L. SNYDER, MD, FACP
Professor, Laboratory Medicine, Yale School of Medicine, Director, Transfusion Medicine Services, Yale New Haven Hospital, New Haven, Connecticut, USA

BRYAN R. SPENCER, PhD
Scientific Affairs, Research Scientist, American Red Cross, Dedham, Massachusetts, USA

PHILIP C. SPINELLA, MD, FCCM
Department of Pediatrics, Division of Pediatric Critical Care Medicine, Washington University School of Medicine, St Louis, Missouri, USA

MICHAEL B. STREIFF, MD
Professor of Medicine and Pathology, Division of Hematology, Department of Medicine, Johns Hopkins University School of Medicine, Baltimore, Maryland, USA

DAVID F. STRONCEK, MD
Center for Cellular Engineering, Department of Transfusion Medicine, Clinical Center, National Institutes of Health, Bethesda, Maryland, USA

KIMBERLY A. THOMAS, PhD
Department of Pediatrics, Division of Pediatric Critical Care Medicine, Washington University School of Medicine, St Louis, Missouri, USA

DARRELL J. TRIULZI, MD
University of Pittsburgh, Institute for Transfusion Medicine, Pittsburgh, Pennsylvania, USA

STEPHEN J. WAGNER, PhD
Senior Director, Transfusion Innovation Department, American Red Cross Holland Laboratory, Rockville, Maryland, USA

KAMILLE WEST, MD
Section Chief, Blood Services, Department of Transfusion Medicine, Clinical Center, National Institutes of Health, Bethesda, Maryland, USA

GEOFFREY D. WOOL, MD, PhD
Assistant Professor, Department of Pathology, Medical Director of Coagulation Laboratory, The University of Chicago, Chicago, Illinois, USA

Contents

Despite measures to mitigate risk of transfusion-transmitted infections, emerging agents contribute to morbidity and mortality. We outline the epidemiology, risk mitigation strategies, and impact on patients for Zika virus, bacteria, Babesia, and cytomegalovirus. Nucleic acid testing of blood has reduced risk of Zika infection and reduced transfusion-transmitted risk of Babesia. Other collection and testing measures have reduced but not eliminated the risk of sepsis from bacterially contaminated blood components. Cytomegalovirus has almost been eliminated by high-efficiency leukoreduction, but residual transmissions are difficult to distinguish from community-acquired infections and additional antibody testing of blood may confer further safety of susceptible recipients.

In the past 30 years, transfusion safety has increased substantially and blood transfusion is now a safer procedure than at any time in the past. Herein, we provide a comprehensive review of pathogen reduction, which is the new paradigm in transfusion safety. Specifically, we describe the various processes and technologies that are capable of diminishing or neutralizing infectious threats, including those that are not addressed or may not be detected by standard screening techniques. A special emphasis is placed on recent developments that are likely to impact patient care in 2019 and beyond.

Transfusion-related acute lung injury and transfusion-associated circulatory overload are characterized by acute pulmonary edema within 6 hours of blood transfusion. Despite recognition as the leading causes of transfusion-related mortality, they remain difficult to study due to underrecognition and nonspecific diagnostic criteria. Recent study has shown that inflammatory cytokines and cardiopulmonary biomarker may be useful in differentiating pulmonary transfusion reactions and furthering our understanding of their pathogenesis. It is clear that donor / component mitigation and patient blood management strategies have decreased the incidence of pulmonary transfusion reactions. Additional clinical and translational research focused on identifying at-risk transfusion recipients is needed to further prevent these frequently severe cardiopulmonary events.

Iron depletion is a known risk for adult blood donors, but recent studies indicate the prevalence of iron depletion is higher in teenage blood donors. Teenage donors account for more than 10% of the blood collected in the United States and are important for maintaining component availability. Evidence of harm from iron depletion has not been demonstrated, but the area would benefit from further scientific inquiry. Options to protect against iron depletion exist, but each has limitations including cost, logistics, and potential negative impact on blood supply. Blood centers should communicate with donors and make efforts to mitigate these risks.

Novel monoclonal antibody therapies are increasing in number and clinical significance as their role in oncologic formularies expands. Anti-CD38 and anti-CD47/SIRPα agents commonly interfere with pretransfusion compatibility testing. Anti-CD38 interference is mitigated by dithiothreitol, which disrupts CD38 antigen on reagent red cells; however, this modification limits rule-out of all clinically significant antibodies. Several anti-CD47 agents are in clinical trials and demonstrate wide variability in pretransfusion testing interference. Modifications to pretransfusion testing can limit interference by anti-CD47 agents. Rapid dissemination of knowledge of these monoclonal antibody agents to the broader transfusion medicine community is paramount for continued patient transfusion safety.

Red blood cell (RBC) antigen phenotyping is an essential component of transfusion compatibility testing. Serology has been the gold standard method, but its low throughput and risk of diagnostic interference in certain situations limits its applicability. Genotyping is useful for phenotyping in these cases, providing a high-throughput and reliable alternative to serology. Genotyping is indicated in several hematology and oncology patient populations. Because genotyping requires a complex testing environment and bears an additional risk of genotype-phenotype discrepancy, its use is currently limited, but it serves as a useful adjunct and may eventually supplant serology as a new gold standard.

Cell therapies have become an important part of clinical hematology and oncology. Cell therapy laboratories were first established in academic health centers to process ABO-incompatible marrow grafts. These laboratories now produce a wide variety of cell and gene therapies. Some of the most widely used and clinically important cell therapies are T-cell immunotherapies. These therapies include donor lymphocyte infusions, tumor-infiltrating lymphocytes, T-cell receptor–engineered T cells, chimeric antigen receptor T cells, and virus-specific T cells. The clinical application and methods used to manufacture these adoptive cell therapies are reviewed.

J. Wade Atkins, Kamille West, and Kimberly A. Kasow

Cell biology researchers, cellular engineers, and clinicians are teaming together to create powerful drugs. The use of cell-derived products as biologics is rapidly advancing. These human cell–based products have great potential for treating serious conditions but may have unidentified risks. Manipulations, expansions, and gene modifications increase the risks of unexpected outcomes. Implementation of the 21st Century Cures Act is opening avenues for accelerated approvals of these drugs for use in clinical trials and licensure. Although overwhelming, collaboration between regulators, industry, and research and medical communities enables the field to safely meet the needs of critically ill patients.

Steven M. Frank, Shruti Chaturvedi, Ruchika Goel, and Linda M.S. Resar

Providing optimal care to surgical oncology patients who cannot be transfused for religious or other reasons can be challenging. However, with careful planning, using a combination of blood-conserving methods, these "bloodless" patients have clinical outcomes that are similar to other patients who can be transfused. Bloodless surgery can be accomplished safely for most patients, including those undergoing technically challenging oncologic surgery. This article reviews best practices used in a bloodless program during the preoperative, intraoperative, and postoperative periods, with the aim of achieving optimal outcomes when transfusion is not an option for surgical oncology patients.

Thomas G. Scorer, Kristin M. Reddoch-Cardenas, Kimberly A. Thomas, Andrew P. Cap, and Philip C. Spinella

Bleeding related to thrombocytopenia is common in hematology-oncology patients. Platelets stored at room temperature (RTPs) are the current standard of care. Platelets stored in the cold (CSPs) have enhanced hemostatic function relative to RTPs. CSPs were reported to reduce bleeding in hematology-oncology patients. Recent studies have confirmed the enhanced hemostatic properties of CSPs. CSPs may be the better therapeutic option for this population. CSPs may also offer a preferable immune profile, reduced thrombotic risk, and reduced transfusion-transmitted infection risk. The logistical advantages of CSPs would improve outcomes for many patients who currently cannot access platelet transfusions.

HEMATOLOGY/ONCOLOGY CLINICS OF NORTH AMERICA

SERIES OF RELATED INTEREST

Surgical Oncology Clinics of North America
https://www.surgonc.theclinics.com/

THE CLINICS ARE AVAILABLE ONLINE!
Access your subscription at:
www.theclinics.com

Preface

Care of the Patient with Cancer: The Shared Mission of Transfusion Medicine and Hematology/ Oncology

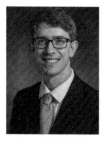
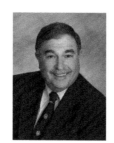

Eric A. Gehrie, MD   Edward L. Snyder, MD, FACP
Editors

The specialties of transfusion medicine and hematology/oncology are closely linked by history as well as by a shared mission to provide outstanding care to patients with blood disorders or cancer. It is not surprising, therefore, that recent advances in transfusion medicine will have a significant impact on the care that hematology/oncology patients receive. Similarly, advances in immunooncology have had a substantial impact on transfusion medicine laboratory operations. In this issue of *Hematology/ Oncology Clinics of North America*, we present articles that highlight some of the most recent and impactful developments in transfusion medicine, with an emphasis on advances in patient safety, cellular therapy, and patient blood management. They are all focused on how recent advances in transfusion medicine improve the care of the hematology/oncology patient.

Spotlighting patient safety, this issue begins with an update on existing as well as emerging blood-borne pathogens. This article is followed by a discussion of the pathogen reduction technologies that aim to diminish the infectious potential of viruses, bacteria, and parasites that could contaminate a donated unit of blood or components. The subsequent articles focus on noninfectious hazards associated with blood, including TACO (transfusion- related circulatory overload) and TRALI (transfusion-related acute lung injuries) among vulnerable hematology/oncology transfusion recipients. Iron deficiency anemia in blood donors is also addressed. The latter article may be of particular interest to the hematologist, as potential new regulatory requirements regarding ferritin monitoring among blood donors, if implemented, may lead to an increase in hematology consultations for healthy blood donors once they are informed

Hematol Oncol Clin N Am 33 (2019) xiii–xiv
https://doi.org/10.1016/j.hoc.2019.06.001
0889-8588/19/© 2019 Published by Elsevier Inc.

by their blood center that they are iron deficient due to frequent blood donation. Next, the focus shifts to both innate and acquired recipient factors that impact the ability of the blood bank to provide crossmatch-compatible blood for hematology/oncology patients, many of whom are chronically anemic and are in need of frequent red cell transfusions. Within this topic, special emphasis is placed on the limits of the serologic crossmatch among patients undergoing treatment with monoclonal antibody therapy or patients with variations in genes that control minor red cell antigen expression.

Cellular therapy has been an area of enormous promise and growth within oncology, and the impact of this treatment modality has been clearly appreciated in the blood bank, as well. This special issue includes an article highlighting recent advances in T-cell immunotherapeutics, followed by an update on the latest regulatory standards that will impact the policies and practices of cell therapy programs both today and in the future.

The final articles of the special issue focus on the rapidly growing field of patient blood management. The most successful patient blood management programs are truly multidisciplinary, and thus, we include sections focusing on perioperative management, new trends in the treatment of acute bleeding, coagulation factor stewardship, and pediatrics.

Taken together, we hope that these articles will provide a timely update on the efforts that the field of transfusion medicine is undertaking to provide support to hematology and oncology service lines. We believe that the future is bright, not only with regard to new and emerging therapeutics but also for continued collaboration between transfusion medicine and hematology/oncology specialists.

Eric A. Gehrie, MD
Pathology and Surgery
The Johns Hopkins Medical Institutions
1800 Orleans Street
Zayed Tower, Suite 3081A
Baltimore, MD 21287, USA

Edward L. Snyder, MD, FACP
Laboratory Medicine
Yale University School of Medicine
20 York Street, PS 329C
New Haven, CT 06520, USA

E-mail addresses:
egehrie1@jhmi.edu (E.A. Gehrie)
edward.snyder@yale.edu (E.L. Snyder)

Existing and Emerging Blood-Borne Pathogens

Impact on the Safety of Blood Transfusion for the Hematology/Oncology Patient

Stephen J. Wagner, PhD[a],*, David A. Leiby, PhD[b],
John D. Roback, MD, PhD[c]

KEYWORDS

- Zika virus • Bacteria • Sepsis • Cytomegalovirus • Babesia • Babesiosis
- Transfusion-transmitted

KEY POINTS

- Transfusion-transmitted bacterial sepsis occurs most frequently from platelet transfusions and can result in significant morbidity and mortality.
- The risk of transfusion-transmitted bacterial sepsis is reduced by careful cleansing of the phlebotomy site, sample diversion of the first aliquot of collected blood, and bacterial testing.
- Transfusion-transmitted babesiosis poses a significant risk for hematology and oncology patients, causing a spectrum of disease and potentially leading to severe medical complications.
- The risk of acquiring transfusion-transmitted babesiosis can be mitigated by transfusing blood products, especially red cells, that have been screened for *Babesia* using a licensed blood donor screening assay.
- Whether TT-CMV (still) occurs in the setting of nearly universal leukoreduction is controversial, but if additional measures are required, providing units that are also CMV-negative has been highly effective at preventing CMV transmission in low-birthweight neonates.

Disclosure: This work reflects the views of the authors and should not be construed to represent FDA's views or policies. S.J. Wagner is a member of the BioMérieux, Inc., scientific advisory board. D.A. Leiby and J.D. Roback have nothing to disclose.
^a Transfusion Innovation Department, American Red Cross Holland Laboratory, 15601 Crabbs Branch Way, Rockville, MD 20855, USA; ^b Division of Emerging & Transfusion Transmitted Diseases, FDA/CBER/OBRR, 10903 New Hampshire Avenue, Building 71, Room 4044, Silver Spring, MD 20993, USA; ^c Department of Pathology and Laboratory Medicine, Emory University School of Medicine, EUH D-655, 1364 Clifton Road NE, Atlanta, GA 30322, USA
* Corresponding author.
E-mail address: stephen.wagner@redcross.org

ZIKA VIRUS

Zika is a positive-sense, 10.7-kb enveloped flavivirus (ZIKV) first isolated in a rhesus monkey in 1947 in the Zika Forest of Uganda.[1] Early recognized infections in Africa and South Asia were associated with a febrile rash illness.[2] In 2007 and 2013, larger outbreaks occurred in Yap Island, Federated States of Micronesia, and French Polynesia, respectively.[3,4] Later, an association of ZIKV infection and a 20-fold increase in Guillain-Barré syndrome in French Polynesia was recognized.[5] Cases of ZIKV were first observed in Brazil in 2015,[6] and additional infections that year were linked geographically and temporally to an increased rate of microcephaly of infants born from infected mothers.[7] Since its introduction in Brazil, ZIKV has spread to many countries in Latin America and the Caribbean.[8]

The primary vector for ZIKV transmission in the Americas is the *Aedes aegypti* mosquito, whose range includes the southern region of the continental United States.[9] Among the 5724 cases of ZIKV in the continental United States, most infections (5448) have been associated with travel to endemic areas, 231 were presumed to be caused by local mosquito-borne transmission, and the remainder were thought to be caused by sexual transmission (55 cases) and other causes.[10] The autochthonous vector-borne cases occurred in 2 counties each in South Florida and South Texas.

ZIKV that is transmitted from mother to fetus may result in fetal loss, a spectrum of neurologic syndromes, and microcephaly.[11] The risk of microcephaly seems to be greatest during the first trimester, although microencephaly has been observed by infections acquired during all 3 trimesters.[12] Rates of microcephaly in Brazil ranged from 0.88% to 13% depending on underlying assumptions of the infection rate.[12]

ZIKV can be transmitted by blood transfusion based on published reports of 3 transmissions observed in Brazil,[13,14] and circulating ZIKV RNA was detected in 2.8% of blood donors in French Polynesia.[15] Approximately 80% of ZIKV cases are asymptomatic,[16] making infection diagnosis by physical examination before phlebotomy unlikely. Symptoms in adults usually resolve within 1 week.[3,4] Based on the potential for transmission of an arthropod-borne disease of serious consequences by blood transfusion, the US Food and Drug Administration (FDA) provided guidance for reducing the risk of ZIKV transmission by recommending individual nucleic acid testing of all US blood donors.[17,18] In June 2016, the American Red Cross implemented a primary test for ZIKV RNA by using transcription-meditated amplification (TMA) of plasma samples, and confirmatory tests by repeat TMA of plasma and red cell samples, exploratory minipool testing (rather than individual testing), real-time reverse-transcriptase polymerase chain reaction, and immunoglobulin M (IgM) serologic testing.[19] Between June 2016 and September 2017, 3,932,176 donations were tested by TMA with 160 initially reactive, and 9 confirmed positive. Six of the 9 were repeat reactive with TMA and 4 of the 6 were IgM negative, suggesting window period infection. Three of the 4 samples representing window period infections could be detected by minipool TMA; the remaining sample could not be tested. Two of the 9 confirmed positive donations were autochthonous vector-borne cases in Florida, 6 infections were likely acquired by travel to endemic areas, and 1 donor received an experimental ZIKV vaccine.

It was estimated that the cost of identifying the 8 mosquito-borne ZIKV infections in US donors was $41.7 million.[19] In 2018, the FDA announced new guidance for ZIKV testing, moving away from testing each individual donation to testing pooled donations.[20]

BACTERIA

Bacterial contamination of blood and sepsis on transfusion has long been recognized for morbidity and mortality to recipients, including hematology and oncology patients.[21] Although bacteria can either be present in whole blood or introduced via the skin during phlebotomy, more bacterial species can proliferate and ultimately cause sepsis in the room temperature conditions used for platelet storage than the refrigerated conditions used for red cell storage. Organisms identified with red cell-associated bacterial sepsis often involve psychrophilic species capable of growth at 1°C to 6°C.[22–24] Red cell-associated bacterial sepsis occurs with an estimated frequency of 1 in 2.8 million units (passive reporting). (Dy B. American Red Cross Hemavigilance Program (2004-2018), personal communication, 11/15/2018, W. SJ, Editor. 2018.) Sepsis in platelet recipients with recorded symptoms occurs in approximately 1 of 10,000 units in studies using active surveillance and roughly 1 in 100,000 units in studies reliant on passive surveillance.[25,26]

Estimated bacterial loads in contaminated units at collection are hypothesized to be extremely low; 1 case of sepsis was observed in only 1 unit derived from a triple apheresis collection in which the sister units were uncontaminated.[27] Bacteria proliferate in some of these units to high levels; most cases of sepsis in platelet recipients with recorded symptoms involve units that contain greater than 10^5 colony-forming units (CFUs)/mL bacteria.[28] Symptoms of transfusion-associated bacterial sepsis include fever, severe chills, rigors, hypotension, tachycardia, nausea and vomiting, dyspnea, circulatory collapse, or intravascular coagulation within 24 hours of transfusion. If symptoms are recognized during transfusion, the transfusion should be immediately stopped, medical care administered, and an investigation for transfusion-associated sepsis begun, including culture of residual platelets and patient blood.[29] Transfusion-associated bacterial sepsis should be considered in the diagnosis of patients exhibiting septic signs up to 24 hours following transfusion.[25]

Several modifications in the collection and testing of platelets have been made to diminish septic risk. Cleansing of the antecubital fossa reduces contamination of platelets by skin-derived organisms and depends on the types of disinfectants and methods used.[30,31] Diversion of the initial volume of whole blood away from the primary collection container to a separate pouch removes bacteria present in skin plugs caused by coring of skin during collection, diminished true-positives in platelet bacterial culture by 41% to 76%[26,30,32] and reduced sepsis from whole blood-derived platelet pools by approximately 10-fold.[32]

Early culturing efforts used 4- to 5-mL samples taken 24 to 36 hours postcollection.[33,34] Recognition that many contaminated platelets were missed owing to sampling error (no bacteria in the small sample volume but bacteria in the platelet container)[35] led to increasing sample volume to 8 to 10 mL and resulted in a 74% decline of septic events when coupled with sample diversion.[36,37] Still, culture detection is predicted to be less than 40%.

Efforts have been focused to investigate secondary testing methods. One FDA-approved method uses lateral flow assay of platelet extracts with antibody detection of Gram-positive and Gram-negative bacterial cell wall components and has a detection sensitivity of 10^3 to 10^5 CFUs/mL.[38] Clinical use of the test detected 9 true-positive platelet units of 27,620 primary culture-negative units.[39] The false-positive rate was 0.5%. The test allows extension of platelet shelf life to up to 7 days storage in approved platelet products.

Other secondary detection strategies involve culturing. One study by Bloch and colleagues[40] performed hospital-based aerobic culturing on day 3 using 5-mL samples. Platelets were transfused up to day 5 with no quarantine postinoculation. Of 23,044 culture-negative apheresis platelets initially sampled on day 1, secondary culture on day 3 yielded 5 true-positive test results. No septic reactions were observed during the 13-month study compared with 3 definite and 4 possible cases in the preceding year. Another study involved secondary culture performed on day 4 using 8 mL each in aerobic and anaerobic bottles.[41] Platelets were stored up to 7 days and not quarantined following secondary culture. Using this strategy, there were 5 true-positives of 51,041 platelets that were culture-negative on day 1.[42] Finally, researchers have evaluated increasing the volume and sampling time to improve the sensitivity of primary culture.[43] The use of secondary testing, improved primary culture, or pathogen reduction (see Eric A. Gehrie and colleagues' article, "Pathogen Reduction: The State of the Science in 2019," in this issue) promises to decrease septic risk from platelet transfusions.

BABESIA

Babesia spp are intraerythrocytic protozoan parasites and the causative agents of babesiosis in animals and humans. Infections are transmitted naturally by hard-bodied tick vectors, often of the family Ixodidae. Although most human cases of babesiosis are attributable to *B microti*, infections have also been ascribed to *B divergens*, *B duncani*, and *B venatorum*.[44] The first human infection was reported in 1957, near present day Zagreb, Croatia, in a 33-year-old splenectomized tailor exposed to *B divergens*.[45] In the United States, the index case occurred in a 46-year-old splenectomized California man in 1966; however, the infecting *Babesia* species was unconfirmed. The first US case attributed to *B microti* was reported on Nantucket Island, Massachusetts, in 1969. Since this initial identification, the geographic range of *B microti* has expanded and the parasite is now endemic throughout the Northeast and Upper Midwest, causing approximately 2000 babesiosis cases annually in the United States. With its rapid emergence and recognition as a growing public health concern, babesiosis became nationally notifiable in 2011.

Babesial infections in humans demonstrate a spectrum of disease, ranging from asymptomatic to severe, including fatalities.[46] Asymptotic infections are common among immunocompetent persons who may not recognize infection or experience only mild nonspecific symptoms (eg, cold, flu-like) that resolve spontaneously. More severe cases of babesiosis seem to be associated with neonates/infants, the elderly, immunocompromised, and especially asplenic patients in whom parasitemias may approach 85%. When present, symptoms appear 1 to 4 weeks postinfection and include fever, headache, chills, myalgia, malaise, drenching sweats, and hemolytic anemia. Susceptible populations may exhibit more serious complications consisting of hemodynamic instability, acute respiratory distress, severe hemolysis, disseminated intravascular coagulation, renal dysfunction, hepatic compromise, myocardial infarction, and death. In most instances symptomatic infections with demonstrable parasitemia are effectively treated with clindamycin/quinine or atovaquone/azithromycin.[47] In rare cases, severe anemia due to high parasitemia may require emergency exchange transfusion to rapidly reduce parasitemia and associated anemia.

In addition to vector-borne transmission, *Babesia* can also be transmitted by solid organ transplantation and transfusion of blood obtained from *Babesia*-infected donors. The first case of transfusion-transmitted babesiosis (TTB) occurred in Boston, Massachusetts, during 1979 and implicated a *B microti*-infected donor from Nantucket Island. A comprehensive report from the Centers for Disease Control and Prevention (CDC) published in 2011 described 162 US cases of TTB, indicating a rapid rise in cases over a 30-year period.[48] Indeed, anecdotal evidence suggests the current number of cases of TTB exceeds 200. Except for 3 cases attributed to *B duncani*, all other cases have implicated *B microti*. Clinical features in cases of TTB are like those observed for vector-borne infections; however, symptoms may not appear until

9 weeks posttransfusion; longer incubation periods have been observed among patients with sickle cell disease.[49] Implicated components were almost exclusively red cells, including those cryopreserved, but at least 4 cases have involved random donor platelets. No cases have implicated apheresis platelets or plasma. Among the 162 cases of TTB described by the CDC, 28 resulted in fatalities caused in part by babesiosis.

An extensive review of underlying medical conditions in TTB recipients revealed infections in patients with hematologic disease and solid tumors.[50] Among 165 confirmed cases of TTB, the underlying disease was identified for 93 (56%). TTB was reported to occur in a wide variety of conditions including 31 (19%) hematologic and 8 (5%) associated with solid tumors. Among patients with underlying hematologic disease, 10 of 31 (6%) were reported to have hematologic malignancy and 17 had benign disease, which included 9 patients with sickle cell disease; 4 patients could not be characterized. Death occurred in 32 (19%) of the patients with TTB, and babesiosis was identified as the cause in 25 cases. Four deaths were reported in patients with hematologic disease, and 1 death was associated with a solid tumor. In general, cases of TTB were reported to occur across all age groups demonstrating a variety of underlying conditions.

Several blood disorders (eg, sickle cell, thalassemia) may pose increased risk for babesiosis due to chronic transfusion and misdiagnosis. Extended incubation periods in patients with sickle cell disease were described earlier; however, for some cases of TTB the correct diagnosis may be delayed by misinterpretation of observed symptoms. For example, in some chronically transfused patients with sickle cell disease, development of hemolytic anemia may initially be attributed to the development of alloantibodies and autoantibodies, thereby obscuring an underlying *B microti* infection.[51] A case of TTB involving *B duncani* posed similar diagnostic challenges because the patient demonstrated multicause anemia.[52] In these instances, treatment may be delayed pending the correct diagnosis, often due to a fortuitous blood smear. Chronically transfused patients with thalassemia are also at increased risk for infection. A recent report from the CDC identified *Babesia* among thalassemia patients with exposure to potentially transfusion-associated infectious diseases.[53]

When devising strategies to mitigate TTB in hematology and oncology patients, several factors need to be considered, largely associated with risk. Patients at greatest risk are those receiving blood products collected in *Babesia*-endemic areas of the Northeast and Upper Midwest. As discussed previously, almost all cases of TTB have implicated red cells, but several cases involved whole blood-derived platelets. As *B microti* resides intraerythrocytically, leukoreduced blood products do not prevent transmission, nor does irradiation. Since 2012, the American Red Cross has prospectively screened blood donations in areas endemic for *B microti*, first under Investigational New Drug and later using licensed blood screening assays (ie, arrayed fluorescence immunoassay and real-time polymerase chain reaction).[54] During the testing period (June 2012–May 2018), no cases of TTB were associated with 506,540 screened donations from Connecticut, Massachusetts, Minnesota, and Wisconsin. However, during this same period, 23 cases of TTB were associated with 1,163,607 unscreened donations collected in Connecticut and Massachusetts. An alternative approach is to selectively provide screened units to at-risk patient groups (ie, neonates, pediatric patients with sickle cell disease or thalassemia).[55] Thus, blood donation screening for *B microti* seems to effectively mitigate TTB risk. Although the originally approved screening assays were withdrawn from the market in November 2018, the FDA approved a *Babesia* nucleic acid test (NAT) for blood donor screening in January 2019, which should prevent TTB. As discussed in Drs Eric A. Gehrie and colleagues' article, "Pathogen Reduction: The State of the Science in 2019," in this issue, pathogen reduction provides an alternative to blood screening, but pathogen reduction has only been approved for apheresis platelets and plasma, not red cell products which represent the greatest risk for transmitting *Babesia*.

CYTOMEGALOVIRUS

Cytomegalovirus (CMV) generates an inordinate amount of debate in transfusion medicine. In fact, one of the few areas of agreement between experts is that CMV infection can cause serious disease and even death in an immunocompromised patient. Virtually every other question is contentious: (1) Is infectious CMV transmitted by transfusion? (2) Is leukoreduction (LR) by itself effective at eliminating the risks of transfusion-transmitted CMV (TT-CMV)? (3) Are there advantages to combining leukoreduction with CMV serology? (4) Is there a role for CMV NAT? For completeness, there is one more issue that unifies CMV experts: once universal pathogen reduction is implemented, these debates will (finally) be over.

The first issue is surprisingly contentious. Some have argued that there is no strong evidence for infectious CMV transmission by transfusion.[56] On the other hand, a large number of studies support the occurrence of TT-CMV, particularly decades ago before (nearly) universal leukoreduction was the norm (reviewed in Vamvakas[57]). It is unclear whether this issue will ever be resolved, in part because the relatively high rate of community-acquired CMV infection (estimated at 1% of the population per year) always presents a readily available alternative explanation for cases of presumed TT-CMV. Viral genotyping could be used to obtain more definitive evidence, but this approach has not yet been applied in a comprehensive fashion to address the occurrence of TT-CMV. A given practitioner's opinion on whether TT-CMV occurs or not often influences their position on the next question.

The second issue is also contentious, although less of a surprise. For over 20 years, the efficacy of LR for the prevention of TT-CMV has been repeatedly investigated. These are large, complex, and expensive studies. Moreover, the results of early work[58] are difficult to translate to the modern era because of significant advancements in LR methodologies. Nonetheless, some practitioners who believe TT-CMV no longer occurs, as well as some large national blood systems (eg, Canadian Blood Service [CBS]), have deemed LR alone as the default approach to preventing TT-CMV. This decision relies heavily on a recent statistical analysis of the risks of TT-CMV, the percentage of CMV-infected monocytes in the peripheral blood of donors, and the odds of LR failure.[59] Unfortunately, as the authors acknowledge, their analysis required some assumptions for which solid data are lacking. For example, they assume that cell-free CMV in the plasma (which can be found at high levels shortly after infection) is not infectious to a transfusion recipient. Nonetheless, as some prospective studies have shown, any residual risk of CMV transmission with LR-only units is probably quite low.[60]

The third question that comes up is whether an additional safety margin can be gained by combining CMV serology with LR. American neonatologists with whom the author has worked with clearly believe in this approach. For example, when we set out to perform a large randomized controlled trial of CMV serology versus LR-only, they were unwilling to participate initially because they continue to insist that their at-risk patients receive LR- and CMV-seronegative units. Although one can debate the scientific underpinnings of this decision, as discussed above, the results of our modified study (a prospective longitudinal analysis of CMV transmission in CMV-seronegative low-birthweight neonates who received CMV-seronegative and LR units) clearly showed that this approach was extremely safe.[61] No cases of TT-CMV were found following transfusion of 2061 CMV-seronegative LR units. Interestingly, CBS also allows CMV serology to be used in conjunction with LR for transfusions given to the youngest of patients (fetuses receiving intrauterine transfusion).

To understand the interest in the fourth issue, why CMV NAT may be a useful addition to LR (and could be superior to using CMV serology), consider the point raised above: does LR effectively interdict free virus in plasma? The highest titer of free virus occurs during the early phases of infection, much of it before seroconversion. So if infectious CMV in the plasma of a newly infected blood donor passed through the filter into the unit, the unit could be infectious but not detected by CMV serology. However, with a sufficiently sensitive CMV NAT assay, plasma-free virus could be identified, and that unit could be removed from inventory. This is an area of current investigation.

For the sake of completeness, methods of pathogen inactivation that are either FDA approved, or are going through the approval process, are highly effective at preventing TT-CMV, at least in murine models.[62,63] Thus, at some point in the future, after implementation of universal pathogen reduction, we may stop debating the significance of TT-CMV, even though many of the questions raised could still remain.

REFERENCES

1. Dick GW, Kitchen SF, Haddow AJ. Zika virus. I. Isolations and serological specificity. Trans R Soc Trop Med Hyg 1952;46(5):509–20.
2. Simpson DI. Zika virus infection in man. Trans R Soc Trop Med Hyg 1964;58:335–8.
3. Lanciotti RS, Kosoy OL, Laven JJ, et al. Genetic and serologic properties of Zika virus associated with an epidemic, Yap State, Micronesia, 2007. Emerg Infect Dis 2008;14(8):1232–9.
4. Cao-Lormeau VM, Roche C, Teissier A, et al. Zika virus, French Polynesia, South Pacific, 2013. Emerg Infect Dis 2014;20(6):1085–6.
5. Oehler E, Watrin L, Larre P, et al. Zika virus infection complicated by Guillain-Barre syndrome–case report, French Polynesia, December 2013. Euro Surveill 2014;19(9) [pii:20720].
6. Zanluca C, Melo VC, Mosimann AL, et al. First report of autochthonous transmission of Zika virus in Brazil. Mem Inst Oswaldo Cruz 2015;110(4):569–72.
7. Brazilian government (Brazil), M.d.S., Ministério da Saúde divulga boletim epidemiológico sobre microcefalia 2015. Available at: http://www.brasil.gov.br/noticias/saude/2015/11/ministerio-da-saude-divulga-boletim-epidemiologico-sobre-micro cefalia. Accessed June 19, 2019.
8. Hennessey M, Fischer M, Staples JE. Zika virus spreads to new areas - region of the Americas, May 2015-January 2016. MMWR Morb Mortal Wkly Rep 2016; 65(3):55–8.
9. Centers for Disease Control and Prevention. Estimated potential range of Aedes aegypti and Aedes albopictus in the United States. Atlanta (GA): Centers for Disease Control and Prevention; 2017.
10. Centers for Disease Control and Prevention. Cumulative Zika virus disease case counts in the United States, 2015-2018. Atlanta (GA): Centers for Disease Control and Prevention; 2018.
11. Franca GV, Schuler-Faccini L, Oliveira WK, et al. Congenital Zika virus syndrome in Brazil: a case series of the first 1501 livebirths with complete investigation. Lancet 2016;388(10047):891–7.
12. Johansson MA, Mier-y-Teran-Romero L, Reefhuis J, et al. Zika and the risk of microcephaly. N Engl J Med 2016;375(1):1–4.

13. Barjas-Castro ML, Angerami RN, Cunha MS, et al. Probable transfusion-transmitted Zika virus in Brazil. Transfusion 2016;56(7):1684–8.
14. Motta IJ, Spencer BR, Cordeiro da Silva SG, et al. Evidence for transmission of Zika virus by platelet transfusion. N Engl J Med 2016;375(11):1101–3.
15. Musso D, Nhan T, Robin E, et al. Potential for Zika virus transmission through blood transfusion demonstrated during an outbreak in French Polynesia, November 2013 to February 2014. Euro Surveill 2014;19(14) [pii:20761].
16. Duffy MR, Chen TH, Hancock WT, et al. Zika virus outbreak on Yap Island, Federated States of Micronesia. N Engl J Med 2009;360(24):2536–43.
17. Food and Drug Administration. Donor screening recommendations to reduce the risk of transmission of Zika virus by human cells, tissues, and cellular and tissue-based products. Silver Spring (MD): Food and Drug Administration; 2016.
18. Food and Drug Administration. Revised recommendations for reducing the risk of Zika virus transmission by blood and blood components. Silver Spring (MD): Food and Drug Administration; 2016.
19. Saa P, Proctor M, Foster G, et al. Investigational testing for Zika virus among U.S. Blood donors. N Engl J Med 2018;378(19):1778–88.
20. Food and Drug Administration. FDA announces revised guidance on the testing of donated blood and blood components for Zika virus. Silver Spring (MD): Food and Drug Administration; 2018.
21. Goldman M, Blajchman MA. Blood product-associated bacterial sepsis. Transfus Med Rev 1991;5(1):73–83.
22. Leclercq A, Martin L, Vergnes ML, et al. Fatal *Yersinia enterocolitica* biotype 4 serovar O:3 sepsis after red blood cell transfusion. Transfusion 2005;45(5):814–8.
23. Tabor E, Gerety RJ. Five cases of pseudomonas sepsis transmitted by blood transfusions. Lancet 1984;1(8391):1403.
24. Roth VR, Arduino MJ, Nobiletti J, et al. Transfusion-related sepsis due to *Serratia liquefaciens* in the United States. Transfusion 2000;40(8):931–5.
25. Hong H, Xiao W, Lazarus HM, et al. Detection of septic transfusion reactions to platelet transfusions by active and passive surveillance. Blood 2016;127(4):496–502.
26. Eder AF, Kennedy JM, Dy BA, et al. Limiting and detecting bacterial contamination of apheresis platelets: inlet-line diversion and increased culture volume improve component safety. Transfusion 2009;49(8):1554–63.
27. Kaufman RM, Savage WJ. *Staphylococcus aureus* sepsis from one cocomponent of a "triple" apheresis platelet donation. Transfusion 2014;54(7):1704.
28. Jacobs MR, Good CE, Lazarus HM, et al. Relationship between bacterial load, species virulence, and transfusion reaction with transfusion of bacterially contaminated platelets. Clin Infect Dis 2008;46(8):1214–20.
29. Eder AF, Goldman M. How do I investigate septic transfusion reactions and blood donors with culture-positive platelet donations? Transfusion 2011;51(8):1662–8.
30. de Korte D, Curvers J, de Kort WL, et al. Effects of skin disinfection method, deviation bag, and bacterial screening on clinical safety of platelet transfusions in the Netherlands. Transfusion 2006;46(3):476–85.
31. Benjamin RJ, Dy B, Warren R, et al. Skin disinfection with a single-step 2% chlorhexidine swab is more effective than a two-step povidone-iodine method in preventing bacterial contamination of apheresis platelets. Transfusion 2011;51(3):531–8.
32. Robillard P, Delage G, Itaj NK, et al. Use of hemovigilance data to evaluate the effectiveness of diversion and bacterial detection. Transfusion 2011;51(7):1405–11.

33. Su LL, Kamel H, Custer B, et al. Bacterial detection in apheresis platelets: blood systems experience with a two-bottle and one-bottle culture system. Transfusion 2008;48(9):1842–52.

34. Eder AF, Kennedy JM, Dy BA, et al. Bacterial screening of apheresis platelets and the residual risk of septic transfusion reactions: the American Red Cross experience (2004-2006). Transfusion 2007;47(7):1134–42.

35. Wagner SJ, Eder AF. A model to predict the improvement of automated blood culture bacterial detection by doubling platelet sample volume. Transfusion 2007; 47(3):430–3.

36. Fang CT, Chambers LA, Kennedy J, et al. Detection of bacterial contamination in apheresis platelet products: American Red Cross experience, 2004. Transfusion 2005;45(12):1845–52.

37. Benjamin RJ, Dy B, Perez J, et al. Bacterial culture of apheresis platelets: a mathematical model of the residual rate of contamination based on unconfirmed positive results. Vox Sang 2014;106(1):23–30.

38. Vollmer T, Hinse D, Kleesiek K, et al. The Pan Genera Detection immunoassay: a novel point-of-issue method for detection of bacterial contamination in platelet concentrates. J Clin Microbiol 2010;48(10):3475–81.

39. Jacobs MR, Smith D, Heaton WA, et al. Detection of bacterial contamination in prestorage culture-negative apheresis platelets on day of issue with the Pan Genera Detection test. Transfusion 2011;51(12):2573–82.

40. Bloch EM, Marshall CE, Boyd JS, et al. Implementation of secondary bacterial culture testing of platelets to mitigate residual risk of septic transfusion reactions. Transfusion 2018;58(7):1647–53.

41. Murphy WG, Foley M, Doherty C, et al. Screening platelet concentrates for bacterial contamination: low numbers of bacteria and slow growth in contaminated units mandate an alternative approach to product safety. Vox Sang 2008; 95(1):13–9.

42. Food and Drug Administration. Blood products advisory meeting. Transcripts. Silver Spring (MD): Food and Drug Administration; 2018. Available at: https://www.fda.gov/downloads/AdvisoryCommittees/CommitteesMeetingMaterials/Blood VaccinesandOtherBiologics/BloodProductsAdvisoryCommittee/UCM618508.pdf. Accessed July 18, 2018.

43. McDonald C, Allen J, Brailsford S, et al. Bacterial screening of platelet components by National Health Service Blood and Transplant, an effective risk reduction measure. Transfusion 2017;57(5):1122–31.

44. Leiby DA. Transfusion-transmitted *Babesia* spp.: bull's-eye on *Babesia microti*. Clin Microbiol Rev 2011;24(1):14–28.

45. Skrabalo Z, Deanovic Z. Piroplasmosis in man; report of a case. Doc Med Geogr Trop 1957;9(1):11–6.

46. Vannier E, Krause PJ. Human babesiosis. N Engl J Med 2012;366(25):2397–407.

47. Krause PJ, Lapore T, Sikand VK, et al. Atovaquone and azithromycin for the treatment of babesiosis. N Engl J Med 2000;343(20):1454–8.

48. Herwaldt BL, Linden JV, Bosserman E, et al. Transfusion-associated babesiosis in the United States: a description of cases. Ann Intern Med 2011;155(8):509–19.

49. Cirino CM, Leitman SF, Williams E, et al. Transfusion-associated babesiosis with an atypical time course after nonmyeloablative transplantation for sickle cell disease. Ann Intern Med 2008;148(10):794–5.

50. Fang DC, McCullough J. Transfusion-transmitted *Babesia microti*. Transfus Med Rev 2016;30(3):132–8.

51. Karkoska K, Louie J, Appiah-Kubi AO, et al. Transfusion-transmitted babesiosis leading to severe hemolysis in two patients with sickle cell anemia. Pediatr Blood Cancer 2018;65(1). https://doi.org/10.1002/pbc.26734.

52. Bloch EM, Herwaldt BL, Leiby DA, et al. The third described case of transfusion-transmitted *Babesia duncani*. Transfusion 2012;52(7):1517–22.

53. Vichinsky E, Neumayr L, Trimble S, et al. Transfusion complications in thalassemia patients: a report from the Centers for Disease Control and Prevention (CME). Transfusion 2014;54(4):972–81 [quiz 971].

54. Tonnetti L, Townsend RL, Deisting BM, et al. The impact of *Babesia microti* blood donation screening. Transfusion 2019;59(2):593–600.

55. Young C, Chawla A, Berardi V, et al. Preventing transfusion-transmitted babesiosis: preliminary experience of the first laboratory-based blood donor screening program. Transfusion 2012;52(7):1523–9.

56. Goldfinger D, Burner JD. You can't get CMV from a blood transfusion: 2017 Emily Cooley award lecture. Transfusion 2018;58(12):3038–43.

57. Vamvakas EC. WBC-containing allogeneic blood transfusion and mortality: a meta-analysis of randomized controlled trials. Transfusion 2003;43(7):963–73.

58. Bowden RA, Slichter SJ, Sayers M, et al. A comparison of filtered leukocyte-reduced and cytomegalovirus (CMV) seronegative blood products for the prevention of transfusion-associated CMV infection after marrow transplant. Blood 1995;86(9):3598–603.

59. Seed CR, Wong J, Polizzotto MN, et al. The residual risk of transfusion-transmitted cytomegalovirus infection associated with leucodepleted blood components. Vox Sang 2015;109(1):11–7.

60. Thiele T, Krüger W, Zimmermann K, et al. Transmission of cytomegalovirus (CMV) infection by leukoreduced blood products not tested for CMV antibodies: a single-center prospective study in high-risk patients undergoing allogeneic hematopoietic stem cell transplantation (CME). Transfusion 2011;51(12):2620–6.

61. Josephson CD, Caliendo AM, Easley KA, et al. Blood transfusion and breast milk transmission of cytomegalovirus in very low-birth-weight infants: a prospective cohort study. JAMA Pediatr 2014;168(11):1054–62.

62. Keil SD, Saakadze N, Bowen R, et al. Riboflavin and ultraviolet light for pathogen reduction of murine cytomegalovirus in blood products. Transfusion 2015;55(4):858–63.

63. Jordan CT, Saakadze N, Newman JL, et al. Photochemical treatment of platelet concentrates with amotosalen hydrochloride and ultraviolet A light inactivates free and latent cytomegalovirus in a murine transfusion model. Transfusion 2004;44(8):1159–65.

Pathogen Reduction
The State of the Science in 2019

Eric A. Gehrie, MD[a], Sara J. Rutter, MD[b], Edward L. Snyder, MD[b],*

KEYWORDS

- Red blood cell transfusion • Platelet transfusion • Plasma transfusion
- Transfusion-transmitted infection • Pathogen reduction • Blood transfusion

KEY POINTS

- Significant improvements in blood collection and donor screening have made blood transfusion safer now than at any point in the past.
- Pathogen reduction is a promising technology that promises to further add to the safety of blood transfusion by diminishing the infectious potential of bacteria, viruses, and parasites that evade donor screening and conventional infectious disease testing.
- There are several different technologies that can be considered types of pathogen reduction. Each technology has slightly different benefits and drawbacks, but not all formulations are equally available in all areas.
- Because oncology patients are often immunosuppressed, they are a key population that stands to benefit from wide availability of pathogen-reduced blood products.

INTRODUCTION

Efforts and processes to ensure safety of the blood supply are critical and widespread in transfusion medicine. Positive patient identification for type and screens and crossmatches, donor exclusions for travel histories to regions endemic for blood-borne pathogens, and donor requirements designed to eliminate human leukocyte antigen (HLA) antibodies from donor plasma are all examples of the transfusion medicine community adapting to new and continuing threats to the blood supply. However, of these concerns, persistent infectious threats pose highly lethal potential dangers.[1]

Disclosure: E.A. Gehrie has performed clinical trials for Cerus Corporation and Terumo BCT. E.L. Snyder has performed clinical trials for Cerus Corporation. S. Rutter has no disclosures to report.
[a] Department of Pathology, Division of Transfusion Medicine, The Johns Hopkins University School of Medicine, 1800 Orleans Street, Zayed Tower Suite 3081A, Baltimore, MD 21287, USA;
[b] Department of Laboratory Medicine, Yale University School of Medicine, 20 York Street, New Haven, CT 06510, USA
* Corresponding author.
E-mail address: Edward.Snyder@yale.edu

The 1980s and 1990s saw an increasing number of cases of blood-borne human immunodeficiency virus (HIV) transmission to hemophiliacs and other transfusion recipients and made the public aware of the infectious risk of blood products via the news headlines on an almost nightly basis.[2,3] Bacterial contamination of blood products, although not as high profile as the HIV crisis, is far more common and continues to be a major threat to the blood supply. Numerous measures have been put in place over the last 40 years in attempts to reduce the risk of transfusion-transmitted infections. Most of these measures have been reactive; that is, implemented after a new pathogen has been recognized and identified. These measures include assays for HIV and hepatitis,[2] and more recently for the Zika and West Nile viruses. However, a growing number of transfusion specialists are questioning the feasibility and practicality of continuing such reactive strategies. Accordingly, attention has turned to more proactive methods: those methods poised to counter a blood-borne pathogen before it has even been identified.[4,5]

A recent example of a proactive approach to control, if not to eradicate, blood-borne pathogens, is pathogen reduction (PR) technology. PR encompasses the use of a variety of reagents and techniques intended to inactivate or reduce pathogens that may be present in a blood product. Various types of PR technologies have been available in Europe for more than 30 years.[6] Although the current US Food and Drug Administration (FDA)–approved methods are designed to treat platelet concentrates, plasma, and coagulation factor concentrates, much work is now being focused on PR techniques applicable to red blood cells (RBCs) and whole blood. A significant amount of literature regarding the safety and efficacy of many of these PR techniques has been published and is discussed in this article.

To discuss the merits and pitfalls of PR blood components, the available technologies must be described first. These are broadly in 2 categories: photoactivated or pH-activated treatments and chemical treatment. Photoactivation techniques applicable to both cellular and plasmatic blood components include psoralen/ultraviolet (UV) A (UVA) therapy, riboflavin/UV light, UVC irradiation alone (without a photosensitizing agent), methylene blue treatment, and quinacrine/glutathione treatment (pH sensitive). Chemical treatment, which is restricted to plasma and factor concentrates, involves use of solvent/detergent (S/D) methods (tri-n-butyl phosphate and octoxynol). S/D techniques are not applicable to cellular blood components because the basis of the technique involves dissolution of the plasma membrane and this would destroy the cellular component.

TECHNOLOGIES
Amotosalen

One method of PR via photoactivation of an added compound is the amotosalen/UVA method. This technique, which can be applied to plasma or platelet concentrates, is currently used in Europe and is also approved by the FDA for use in the United States.[7] PR is achieved by the addition of amotosalen, a psoralen derivative, and activation by UVA light. Psoralens are naturally occurring chemicals and are found in several foods and plants.[8] Amotosalen intercalates into DNA and RNA and, when activated by UVA light, causes covalent cross-linking of those nucleic acids, primarily via pyrimidine binding[5,9]; this prevents replication of pathogens that might be present in the treated product. A compound adsorption device is used to remove excess amotosalen or free photoproducts from the final product.[10] This technique is effective against lipid-enveloped viruses, bacteria, and parasites, as well as many nonenveloped viruses. However, some nonenveloped viruses and spore-forming bacteria have been shown to be resistant to amotosalen/UVA activation and these include hepatitis A virus (HAV) and hepatitis E virus (HEV), parvovirus B19, poliovirus, *Bacillus cereus*, and prions, the agent of variant Creutzfeldt-Jacob disease.[10,11]

PR as a nucleic acid inactivator is much more efficient than gamma radiation. Gamma radiation binds 1 in 37,000 base pairs, whereas the amotosalen/UVA process binds 1 in 87 base pairs.[12] Thus, leukocytes present in platelets treated with the PR technology, like their gamma-irradiated counterparts, are not able to stimulate TA-GVHD.[12–14] Units of PR-treated platelets should not be gamma or x-ray irradiated because this induces more platelet damage without any therapeutic benefit.

Although amotosalen/UVA PR products were FDA approved for use in all populations,[15] there were initial concerns regarding their use in neonates and infants, especially those undergoing blue light phototherapy for hyperbilirubinemia, because of the possibility of residual amotosalen producing a skin rash.[16] Although data on this neonatal population are sparse, recent studies have not shown toxicity or adverse events specifically related to amotosalen/UVA PR in pediatric patients.[17] Another concern for amotosalen/UVA PR regards reports of an increased risk of acute respiratory distress syndrome (ARDS).[11,18,19] Although most reports do not describe ARDS as a problem with transfusion of PR-treated platelets,[19,20] this possibility remains a concern and is the subject of an ongoing INTERCEPT phase IV postmarketing study (PIPER [Phase IV INTERCEPT Platelets Entering Routine Use]).

Amustaline/Glutathione

Unlike platelets and plasma, photochemical PR techniques using psoralens and UVA cannot be effectively applied to RBC units, because hemoglobin absorbs UVA light. In other words, the presence of high concentrations of hemoglobin inhibits cross-linking of psoralens and renders the PR process inefficient, if not ineffective.[21] One system currently under development for RBC units involves treatment with amustaline (S-303) and glutathione. Amustaline is a compound that noncovalently binds and cross-links nucleic acids, neutralizing a large number of potential blood-borne pathogens without relying on ultraviolet light activity.[22]

The decomposition of S-303 is rapid; the half-life is about 25 minutes.[22] Because amustaline may also react with other molecules, a quenching agent, glutathione (GSH), is added as well.[21,22] Although amustaline crosses cell and viral membranes, glutathione does not. Therefore, glutathione is able to neutralize the extracellular effects of amustaline without detracting from the latter's antipathogen activity.

Amustaline is also useful for leukocyte inactivation and prevention of TA-GVHD.[23] Initial studies showed amustaline/GSH-treated RBCs to have similar RBC life span, recovery, and hemoglobin content compared with untreated RBC units; RBC storage characteristics were maintained and were suitable for use over 35 to 42 days of refrigerated storage.[23,24] In addition, a phase III clinical trial showed no difference in RBC usage or patient outcome for amustaline/GSH-treated RBC compared with untreated RBC units.[25] Additional studies are currently underway at several sites to further elucidate the safety and utility of this pathogen inactivation technique. These studies include ReCePI (The study to Evaluate the Efficacy and Safety of the INTERCEPT Blood System for Red Blood Cells in Patients Undergoing Complex Cardiac Surgery Procedures), a phase III randomized clinical trial studying patients undergoing complex cardiovascular surgery in the United States.

Riboflavin

Riboflavin and UV light offer another option for photochemical PR. Riboflavin, otherwise known as vitamin B_2, is recognized by the FDA as a GRAS (generally regarded as safe) compound. As a result, there are few toxicologic concerns associated with its use in PR of blood products.[26,27] This PR technique involves the addition of riboflavin to the blood product and the subsequent illumination of the product with UV light. The riboflavin binds to nucleic acids and, when activated by the illumination step, alters guanine residues via type I and type II redox reactions.[5] This process results in irreversible damage to DNA and RNA, effectively preventing replication.[26,27] In contrast with the amotosalen process, riboflavin does not need to be removed from the product after treatment.[27]

As with amotosalen PR, riboflavin/UV treatment is effective against bacteria, parasites, and enveloped viruses. However, spore-forming bacteria are unaffected by this system. In addition, the riboflavin technique shows activity against some nonenveloped viruses, including HAV and some parvoviruses.[26,27] Again, like amotosalen, riboflavin/UV PR is effective for T-cell inhibition and prevention of TA-GVHD.[26–28] Some studies have also indicated that treatment with riboflavin/UV may decrease the risk of alloimmunization to HLA antigens caused by transfusion.[29,30] However, the risk of RBC antigen alloimmunization does not seem to be affected.[31]

Riboflavin/UV PR systems have not been approved in the United States but are available in Europe and have received the CE (Conformité Européene) mark for use with platelet concentrates, plasma, and whole blood. A phase III randomized clinical trial of riboflavin/UV-treated platelets (MIPLATE [Efficacy of Mirasol-treated Apheresis Platelets in Patients with Hypoproliferative Thrombocytopenia]) is currently underway in the United States.[32]

Ultraviolet C

In addition to the photochemical methods described earlier, illumination of blood components with UVC light alone has also been investigated as a means of PR. This technique solely uses short-wavelength UVC as the pathogen-reducing agent and does not require any additive compounds, which could present a logistical advantage compared with other methods.[33,34] To achieve PR by this method, platelet concentrates must be vigorously agitated while being illuminated by UVC light. This agitation is necessary to ensure that the product is thoroughly mixed and the platelets fully exposed to the UVC light.[33,34] Additional studies on UVC-treated platelets are being conducted.[35,36] UVC PR techniques have been CE marked for platelet concentrates and studies of UVC-treated plasma are underway; UVC PR is not currently available in the United States.

Short-wavelength UVC light induces formation of cyclobutene pyrimidine and pyrimidine-pyrimidone dimers and is known to be bactericidal and viricidal. The technique functions to prevent nucleic acid transcript elongation and stop replication.[37,38] However, UVC light is also known to damage proteins, which poses a barrier to its use for plasma.[33] There may also be effects on platelet function, because some studies have indicated that UVC irradiation can cause platelet aggregation via activation of the $\propto$ II/β3 integrin (GPIIb/IIIa).[39] Other studies have shown varying effects on platelet function caused by differences in UVC dose and plasma content in the platelet concentrates.[33,34] PR using UVC reduces non–spore-forming bacteria by 4 logs; spore-forming bacteria such as B cereus are less affected.[33] This outcome is similar to that seen with other photochemical PR methods. However, viral reduction is considerably more variable with UVC treatment. Nonenveloped viruses, such as HAV and porcine parvovirus (a model for parvovirus B19), are both inactivated by up to 6 logs[37]; enveloped viruses are less predictably reduced. West Nile virus may be reduced by 3.5 to 4 logs, whereas pseudorabies virus (a model for hepatitis B) may be inactivated by only 2 to 3 logs.[33] Of concern is the high degree of resistance shown by HIV-1, which is only reduced by 1 log. There is evidence that retroviruses as a group may be less vulnerable to this PR technique.[33,37,40,41] Some studies have shown that

UVC is active against *Babesia divergens*,[42] but more data on parasite inactivation are needed. The utility of UVC treatment for inactivation of lymphocytes and prevention of TA-GVHD also requires more study, although there is some evidence suggesting that mononuclear cells are inactivated.[43]

UVC has previously been used to treat plasma protein concentrates such as albumin, intravenous immunoglobulin, and factor VIII concentrates.[44,45] Because of the quenching effect of proteins on UVC, higher dose intensity of UVC is required to pathogen reduce plasma. This requirement has hampered the translation of the platform to fresh frozen plasma, although studies are underway to apply such a technique to this blood component.[33,37]

Methylene Blue

Methylene blue (MB) is a phenothiazinium dye that was first developed in 1876 and has found numerous uses over the years, including for treatment of nitrate poisoning, malaria, and methemoglobinemia.[9] MB is known to damage DNA and RNA in the presence of light.[9,46,47]

As such, it has been used as a photosensitizing agent for blood product PR since the early 1990s.[9] MB can intercalate into DNA or bind to the DNA helix, depending on the concentration and ionic strength of Mg^{+2}.[9,26] When exposed to light (peak absorption is at 620–670 nm wavelength), type I (redox) or type II (photo-oxidative) reactions occur, with most of the PR activity resulting from type II reactions.[9,26] After illumination, any remaining MB is removed via filtration.[48,49]

MB treatment is effective for inactivating enveloped viruses and has been noted to have some limited bactericidal action; it does not significantly affect nonenveloped viruses.[9,26,48] Because MB cannot easily penetrate cell membranes, intracellular viruses are also less affected.[9,26] In addition, and in contrast with other photoactivation PR methods, MB treatment does not inactivate leukocytes and has no impact on decreasing the risk of TA-GVHD.[9] Although there seems to be a low degree of toxicity from MB and an overall high safety profile,[47,48] there have been reports of allergic and anaphylactic reactions from MB-treated plasma.[50] As a result, use of MB-treated plasma has been discontinued in some countries.[9,26,51]

Solvent Detergent

S/D treatment of blood products is primarily used for manufacturing PR plasma. The process involves 2 basic steps: pooling a large number of units of plasma, followed by treatment of the pooled blood component. Plasma from up to 1500 donors is pooled according to ABO type.[52] This pooled plasma is filtered using a membrane with a 1-μm pore and subsequently treated with 1% tri(n-butyl) phosphate and 1% octoxynol (Triton X-100) for 60 to 90 minutes.[52] These reagents are then removed by multiple oil and solid phase extractions.[52] In response to ongoing concerns regarding variant Creutzfeldt-Jacob disease transmission from blood products in Europe, a chromatographic process using a specific affinity ligand was added in 2009 to remove any prions present in the plasma.[53,54] Following this step, the plasma is filtered twice and then frozen in 200-mL aliquots.[52] The end result of this process is a highly standardized plasma product, available as A, B, AB, and O products.

S/D plasma's 2 production steps contribute to its PR in 2 distinct ways. First, the S/D treatment disrupts the lipids in viral envelopes,[9] resulting in highly effective inactivation of enveloped viruses, with greater than a 6-log reduction observed.[55] Although bacteria are also inactivated, bacterial contamination of plasma has traditionally been of lesser concern because of the lower risk of bacterial growth in a frozen component. There is also some evidence that S/D treatment leaves intact the bactericidal function of any complement present in the product.[56] Nonenveloped viruses, such as hepatitis A and parvovirus B19, are not affected by S/D treatment.[9,55] Second, the pooling of plasma from numerous donors also confers benefit, because this dilutes the concentration of any pathogens present. This pooling also results in dilution of plasma proteins, which may decrease the risk of allergic reactions and transfusion related acute lung injury.[55,57]

BLOOD COMPONENTS
Whole Blood

Whole blood is again an area of significant current interest in transfusion medicine. Whole blood was the transfusion product of choice in both world wars, as well as in the Vietnam conflict, where it is estimated that 350,000 whole blood units were transfused with a hemolytic transfusion reaction rate of just 1 in 10,000.[58] Beginning in the 1960s with the start of component therapy, whole blood transfusion started to be replaced by component therapy; that is, RBCs, plasma, and platelets, stored in separate bags under storage conditions optimal for each component.

This shift was implemented primarily to facilitate ABO-compatible transfusions because there is no such component as universal-donor whole blood; either the RBCs or the plasma in the whole blood would be incompatible with any non-ABO identical recipient. Furthermore, use of component therapy allows for transfusion of the specific component of interest for patients with isolated anemia, thrombocytopenia, or factor deficiency. Various financial considerations were also present. Most whole blood in the developed world is now converted into components, whereas whole blood remains of interest mainly to the military, select civilian trauma centers, select pediatric cardiac surgery programs, and low-resource regions such as sub-Saharan Africa.[59–64]

In large part because of the desire to provide pathogen-reduced whole blood to low-resource settings where component therapy may not be feasible, a riboflavin and UV light–based platform is currently the most studied whole blood PR formulation in development.[65] In vitro experiments show a multifold inactivation of several clinically relevant pathogens, including *Staphylococcus aureus*, *Yersinia enterocolitica*, *Babesia microti*, *Trypanosoma cruzi*, *Leishmania donovani*, and *Plasmodium falciparum*.[66–70] A clinical trial in Ghana showed a reduction in transfusion-transmitted malaria via whole blood using a system based on riboflavin and UV light.[71] Additional study, including documentation of real-world efficacy against hepatitis B, hepatitis C, and HIV, as well as demonstration of acceptable transfusion outcomes in a variety of settings, is needed to clearly establish the efficacy and feasibility of this system.[72] At present, PR whole blood is not currently available in North America, and the authors are not aware of any pending North American clinical trials.

Red Blood Cells

PR of RBCs is an area of active interest in the United States and internationally, owing to a continued focus on component therapy as opposed to transfusion of whole blood. Studies have been conducted involving RBCs treated with the PR agent amustaline (S-303).[23,25] Several trials of amustaline-treated RBCs are ongoing, including studies of simple RBC transfusions, patients undergoing RBC exchange for sickle cell anemia, and a randomized controlled clinical trial of RBCs transfused to patients undergoing significant cardiac surgery (ReCePI).

Initial studies of amustaline-treated RBCs performed in early 2000 were stopped by the FDA because of the development of positive direct Coombs tests in 2 children with a hemoglobinopathy. After a thorough investigation it was concluded that the children developed weak antibodies to amustaline. This antibody was not associated with any clinical hemolysis. The study was halted but restarted several years later, after the company had evaluated the problem, identified the root cause, and changed the amustaline formulation to minimize the risk of formation of an alloantibody. The concern over development of a positive direct Coombs tests remains, but more data will be accumulated as part of the ReCePI clinical trial. Concerns over the toxicology of amustaline have been addressed in an article by North and colleagues.[22] From a study of the amustaline process, Cancelas and colleagues,[23] and Brixner and colleagues[25] concluded that the PR treatment was compatible with 35-day red cell storage survival and that there was a lack of adverse events. However, riboflavin/UV treatment of red cells showed a significantly shorter acceptable shelf life of 14 to 21 days.[23,25,73,74] More data are needed before conclusions can be drawn. Treatment of RBCs with amustaline is likely to protect against the development of TA-GVHD, because treatment with the compound effectively cross-links DNA base pairs, thus inhibiting lymphocyte viability.

There are no human studies in the United States involving UVC, but there are studies in Europe evaluating this PR technology. The FDA has expressed interest in promoting and fostering blood PR technologies.[75,76] This work will likely spur further laboratory and clinical research on PR technologies.

Platelets

Of the blood products available, platelets are at the highest risk of contamination by bacteria. Thus, PR of platelets is considered to be especially important from a patient safety perspective. Reducing the risk of transfusion-transmitted bacterial infections is a high priority for transfusion medicine for recipient safety. It is also an area of ongoing regulatory oversight.[75,76] At present, the psoralen/UVA light strategy to pathogen reduce platelets is FDA approved in the United States, and a phase IV postmarketing surveillance study (PIPER) is ongoing. The riboflavin/UV-light platform (MIPLATE) is currently enrolling in a multicenter phase III trial in the United States and has been approved for use in Europe since 2007. The UVC light system is further behind in development but may eventually emerge as a viable alternative.[5]

PR platelets are considered to be safe and effective. However, some important concerns remain, such as the impact the PR process may have on posttransfusion platelet counts or residual platelet function. Similar to other product modifications, such as washing and supplementation with platelet additive solution, it is generally accepted that PR systems reduce the degree to which the platelet count is increased by transfusion.[77–79] One study[80] of the riboflavin/UV-light system reported that the corrected count increment (CCI; a measure of posttransfusion platelet increment adjusted for dose and body surface area) in patients transfused with conventional platelets was significantly higher than the CCI of patients transfused with riboflavin-treated platelets (16,939 vs 11,725; $P<.0001$). However, the clinical significance of this finding was unknown, because the study did not identify an obvious signal for increased bleeding risk among the patients transfused with the PR platelets.[80] Similarly, a study of psoralen and UVA light--treated platelets identified that the PR platelets had lower CCIs than patients transfused with conventional platelets, but, again, no difference in bleeding or RBC transfusion was identified.[78] Although data directly comparing the psoralen platform with the riboflavin platform are limited, available information suggests that the 2 technologies are equivalent in terms of hemostatic efficacy.[81]

Ongoing studies will continue to evaluate the hemostatic efficacy as well as the safety of these systems. Importantly, the phase IV study of the amotosalen-treated platelets (PIPER) will provide additional data on the incidence of pulmonary complications associated with their use. There was an early and still controversial concern that amotosalen-treated platelets could contribute to acute lung injury, via an unclear mechanism. This issue was addressed in an article by Corash and colleagues.[19] The investigators' analysis showed no evidence for an association between ARDS and infusion of PR platelets. Similarly, the phase III trial of riboflavin-treated platelets (MIPLATE) will comprehensively assess bleeding outcomes compared with patients transfused with standard platelets.[82] Overall, any detected drawbacks to PR would need to be carefully weighed against the impact of not using pathogen-reduced components, which include a potentially shorter shelf life of platelets as well as an increased risk of transfusion-transmitted disease, including transfusion-transmitted sepsis and emerging pathogens.[83]

Plasma

As mentioned previously, PR of plasma products has been available in Europe for more than 30 years.[6] Many of the efforts to develop a PR plasma component were driven by the realization that HIV and hepatitis were being transmitted via plasma and cryoprecipitate transfusions, especially among patients with hemophilia.[3] For plasma PR, MB treatment and S/D-treated products were among the first to be developed. S/D-treated plasma has been available in the United States in various forms since the 1990s. initially as Plas + S/D distributed by the American Red Cross and more recently as Octaplas manufactured by Octapharma. Newer techniques involving UV-light activation of various compounds represent more recent advances in this field. Of these, only the amotosalen/UVA-based PR system has been approved by the FDA for use in the United States, although it is not widely available.[10]

MB treatment was introduced in the early 1990s[57] and has been shown to be clinically safe.[48,84] This method is active against enveloped viruses, with different degrees of activity against bacteria and nonenveloped viruses; because the dye does not penetrate cell membranes, intracellular viruses and pathogens are not affected.[9,48] However, MB treatment does degrade the quality of the product. Factors V, VIII, XI, protein S, and fibrinogen levels have been shown to be decreased in MB-treated plasma, with significant decreases noted in fibrinogen and factor VIII.[84,85] Measures of activity such as thrombin generation have been shown to be decreased.[86] In addition, other studies have indicated that MB-treated plasma may be inferior to fresh frozen plasma (FFP) when used for treatment of patients with thrombotic thrombocytopenic purpura (TTP) undergoing therapeutic plasma exchange.[87] MB-treated plasma is used in parts of Europe but is not approved for use in the United States.

S/D-treated plasma, which also debuted in Europe in the early 1990s, has been available in several forms over the years. A version that featured a prion elimination step came to the market in 2009.[57] Of note, a previously available S/D-treated plasma product developed in the United States (Plas + S/D) was associated with an increased risk of thromboembolic complications, and it was withdrawn from the market in the early 2000s.[55] This product was manufactured differently from current S/D plasma products,[88] and such adverse events have not been reported with other S/D plasma formulations.[55,89] In the currently available S/D plasma products, levels of most coagulation factors are similar to those in FFP. However, protein S levels are known to be lower in some formulations.[90–92] The lone S/D plasma product (Octaplas) approved by the FDA and available in the United States is available in all ABO types.[93] A so-called universal S/D plasma product in which anti-A and anti-B isohemagglutinins are removed is currently available in Europe. This product can thus be transfused to any patient regardless of blood group.[94,95]

The amotosalen/UVA PR system is also FDA approved for plasma.[10] Several studies have been published showing the safety of this product,[8,96–98] although the package insert does mention a risk for cardiac events.[7] Of note, the research that precipitated this warning was a study of patients with TTP, who may have already been at risk of cardiac involvement because of their disease.[97,99]

Amotosalen treatment may affect the efficacy of plasma, albeit less than MB or S/D-treated products. Amotosalen-treated FFP has similar levels of antithrombotic proteins and coagulation factors as PF24 (plasma frozen within 24 hours).[100] Postthaw levels of labile proteins such as factor V, factor VIII, protein S, and protein C are decreased, with factor VIII showing the greatest decrease.[101] Importantly, although a mild increase in coagulation times of treated units was noted, there has been no indication of a decrease in clinical efficacy.[101] Although fibrinogen levels are maintained in amotosalen-treated plasma,[98] there is evidence that fibrin clot formation is altered in PR-treated plasma, with clots being denser and composed of thinner fibers.[102] The clinical significance of this finding is unclear.

Cryoprecipitate

PR of cryoprecipitate has received less attention than other blood components. Although viral transmission via cryoprecipitate may be a primary concern, the risk of bacterial contamination cannot be disregarded.[103] Despite evidence of continued coagulation factor activity for up to 24 hours after thawing, thawed non-PR cryoprecipitate has a shelf life of only 4 to 6 hours if not transfused.[104] Studies of bacterial growth in thawed cryoprecipitate show that bacteria can multiply to dangerous levels with extended storage times.[103] PR of cryoprecipitate could present an opportunity not just to lessen the risk of bacterial and viral transmission but also to potentially extend the storage (shelf life) of thawed cryoprecipitate.[103]

To that end, several PR methods have been investigated for possible application to cryoprecipitate.[105–107] All such products show varying degrees of protein loss compared with cryoprecipitate made from untreated plasma. Cryoprecipitate from riboflavin-treated plasma showed decreased levels of factor VIII, von Willebrand factor (vWF), and fibrinogen, but still met European standards for cryoprecipitate protein content.[107] Cryoprecipitate from amotosalen-treated plasma showed a decrease in levels of fibrinogen, factor VIII, as well as ADAMTS-13 (a disintegrin and metalloproteinase with a thrombospondin type 1 motif, member 13), whereas levels of vWF were preserved.[105] A comparison of cryoprecipitate from MB-treated plasma and amotosalen-treated plasma found that although both met European standards for content, they also resulted in formation of weaker clots compared with standard cryoprecipitate.[106] Of note, MB-cryoprecipitate contained less factor XIII but significantly more factor VIII than amotosalen-cryoprecipitate.[106] Cryoprecipitate prepared using amotosalen/UVA has the potential to permit room temperature storage up to 5 days postthaw, which may be a significant advancement for centers with populations that could benefit from the rapid provision of large volumes of cryoprecipitate (eg, after tissue plasminogen activator–associated bleeding or postpartum hemorrhage). S/D-treated cryoprecipitate is currently being developed in Europe. In this process, cryoprecipitate is made from non-PR plasma and subsequently undergoes S/D treatment; the resulting product reportedly has good recovery of factor VIII, vWF, and fibrinogen.[108,109]

Factor Concentrates/Derivatives

Although most factor concentrates manufactured are now recombinant, some are made from pooled human plasma. These products are pathogen reduced primarily by treatment with an S/D formulation. S/D treatments can be used because, in the final concentrate, there are no intact cells. Data have shown that S/D-treated factor concentrates are acceptable and safe for clinical use. Because these products are often manufactured from pools of 1000 or more human donors, concentrates untreated by PR technology pose a substantial risk for transmission of blood-borne pathogens.

COMPARATIVE EFFECTIVENESS

As discussed earlier, the major current impetus for the adoption of PR in North America is to mitigate the risk of transfusion-transmitted sepsis. A recent analysis estimated the risk that a platelet concentrate on a hospital blood bank shelf is contaminated with bacteria to be approximately 1:2881.[110] This risk is orders of magnitude higher than the risk of infection transmitted by a virus, such as HIV or hepatitis C, for which donor nucleic acid testing programs are already in place. However, all 3 major PR platforms show promising reduction in most bacteria that are clinically relevant to platelet components, such as S aureus.[59] It is known that bacterial spores are not inactivated by PR.

Regarding viral protection, the amotosalen/UVA and riboflavin/UV platforms show a significant effect against many clinically relevant pathogens, although, similar to the bacterial data, the degree of viral reduction is generally higher using the amotosalen/UVA process. The amotosalen/UVA process has also been shown to be very effective against the chikungunya virus.[111] Importantly, both of these platforms are unable to effectively neutralize small, nonenveloped viruses, and there is a report of transfusion transmission of hepatitis E despite treatment with amotosalen/UVA.[112] Regarding the MB treatment of plasma, it is important to emphasize that this technology has only a small, 1.4-log reduction effect on HIV and there are 2 known cases of HIV transmission despite MB treatment.[59,113] The amotosalen/UVA and the riboflavin/UV platforms have both been found to have significant antiparasite activity against B microti, P falciparum, and T cruzi.[59]

The role of PR in reducing HLA alloimmunization is another area being studied.[114]

COST

PR technology adds cost to the price of a treated component primarily because of the required additional labor and reagent costs during the manufacturing process. Studies have been published evaluating the cost benefit of PR technologies versus traditional methods of ensuring blood component safety, such as bacterial cultures and serologic genetic testing.[115,116] The concern about bacterial contamination of blood products makes PR technology seem more expensive. However, considering the strong likelihood that nonbacterial blood-borne pathogens will appear in the blood supply following movement of these viral or other pathogens out of rural areas where they may be endemic, the cost-effectiveness of PR technology increases significantly. Bacterial cultures, regardless of newer techniques (larger culture volume or longer incubation times) will be ineffective against these new pathogens if they are of viral origin. Further, it will cost millions of dollars to identify new pathogens and develop a suitable detection assay only to have another virus appear soon in a similar fashion. When repeated episodes of new blood-borne pathogens that threaten the existing blood supply are considered, it becomes much more cost-effective to have a PR technology that will proactively interdict these agents. This reality must be considered by the medical community because future blood-borne pathogens are unlikely to be exclusively bacterial. The availability of PR technologies that are effective against viruses, protozoa, spirochetes, and other pathogens thus becomes very cost-effective.[5]

INTEGRATION OF PATHOGEN REDUCED PRODUCTS INTO THE HOSPITAL BLOOD SUPPLY

The integration of PR products into the hospital blood supply can be problematic because of a variety of factors.[117] These factors include the ability of the blood center to supply the treated products in sufficient quantity and with sufficient reliability to support a clinical program. An important task is the need to orient house staff, nursing staff, and various service lines to the use of a new form of a blood product. This orientation also must be done in close cooperation with the information technology department because inability to scan a new blood product into the electronic medical record is a major cause of end-user dissatisfaction. Another major concern is the need to accommodate a dual inventory and to maintain a standard of care that can be justified. Education of the staff before rolling out the PR products, receiving administrative support to pay for the new products, and acceptance by the medical and nursing staff requires an intensive educational effort before the rollout. This process has been described by Rutter and Snyder.[117]

SUMMARY

PR is a burgeoning field of medical research. There are multiple technologies each with their own set of requirements, relative efficacies, and costs. There is no one-size-fits-all solution; currently, each component must be treated separately, which leads to increased cost and decreased availability because of the difficulties with adoption of new manufacturing processes. The importance of developing this technology and encouragement of its use have recently been addressed by the FDA.[75,76] It is clear that a reactive approach of interdicting one new blood-borne pathogen after another is not a feasible or sustainable model.[5] However, only through demonstration of efficiency, increased availability, minimization of toxicity, and a decrease in cost of production will the use of PR achieve widespread use and acceptance.

REFERENCES

1. Schlenk P. Pathogen inactivation technologies for cellular blood components: an update. Transfus Med Hemother 2014;41:309–25.
2. Stramer SL, Dodd RY. Transfusion-transmitted emerging infectious diseases: 30 years of challenges and progress. Transfusion 2014;53:2375–83.
3. Seltsam A. Pathogen inactivation of cellular blood products- an additional safety layer in transfusion medicine. Front Med (Lausanne) 2017;4:219.
4. Stramer SL, Hollinger FB, Katz LM, et al. Emerging infectious disease agents and their potential threat to transfusion safety. Transfusion 2009;49:1S–29S.
5. Snyder EL, Stramer SL, Benjamin RJ. The safety of the blood supply – time to raise the bar. N Engl J Med 2015;372:1882–5.
6. Dumont LJ, Papari M, Aronson CA, et al. Whole-Blood collection and component processing. In: Fung MK, Grossman BJ, Hillyer CD, et al, editors. Technical manual. 18th edition. Bethesda (MD): AABB; 2014. p. 135–61.
7. Cerus Corporation. FDA approves pathogen reduction system to treat platelets. [Press Release]. Available at: http://www.cerus.com/Investors/Press-Releases/Press-Release-Details/2014/FDA-Approves-INTERCEPT-Blood-System-for-Platelets/default.aspx. Accessed June 25, 2019.

8. Lin L, Conlan MG, Tessman J, et al. Amotosalen interactions with platelet and plasma components: absence of neoantigen formation after photochemical treatment. Transfusion 2005;45:1610–20.

9. Pelletier JPR, Transue S, Snyder EL. Pathogen in-activation techniques. Best Pract Res Clin Haematol 2006;19:205–42.

10. Cerus Corporation. INTERCEPT blood system for plasma [package insert] 2015. Concord (CA).

11. Cerus Corporation. INTERCEPT blood system for platelets- small volume processing set [package insert] 2018. Concord (CA).

12. Grass JA, Hei DJ, Metchette K, et al. Inactivation of leukocytes in platelet concentrates by photochemical treatment with psoralen plus UV-A. Blood 1998;91: 2180–8.

13. Luban NL, Drothler D, Moroff G, et al. Irradiation of platelet components: inhibition of lymphocyte proliferation assessed by limiting-dilution analysis. Transfusion 2000;40:348.

14. Pelszynski MM, Moroff G, Luban NL, et al. Effect of gamma irradiation of red blood cell units on T-cell inactivation as assessed by limiting-dilution analysis: implications for preventing transfusion associated graft versus host disease. Blood 1994;83:1683–9.

15. US Food and Drug Administration. Summary of safety and effectiveness data: INTERCEPT blood system for platelets. [Press Release] 2014. Available at: https://www.fda.gov/downloads/BiologicsBloodVaccines/BloodBloodProducts/ApprovedProducts/PremarketApprovalsPMAs/UCM431243.pdf. Accessed June 25, 2019.

16. Jaquot C, Delaney M. Pathogen-inactivated blood products for pediatric patients: blood safety, patient safety, or both? Transfusion 2018;58:2095–101.

17. Schulz W, Gokhale A, McPadden J, et al. Blood utilization and transfusion reactions in pediatric patients transfused with conventional or pathogen reduced platelets. J Pediatr 2019;209:220–5.

18. Snyder E, McCullough J, Slichter SJ, et al. Clinical safety of platelets photochemically treated with amotosalen HCl and ultraviolet A light for pathogen inactivation: the SPRINT trial. Transfusion 2005;45:1864–75.

19. Corash L, Lin JS, Sherman CD, et al. Determination of acute lung injury after repeated platelet transfusions. Blood 2011;117:1014–20.

20. Gokhale A, Schulz W, Bahar B, et al. Transfusion reaction rates of pathogen reduced (PR) vs conventional (CONV) platelets in adults: a single academic center experience [Abstract]. Transfusion 2018;58(S2):111A. Available at: https://onlinelibrary.wiley.com/doi/10.1111/trf.14903.

21. Henschler R, Seifried E, Mufti N. Development of the S-303 pathogen inactivation technology for red blood cell concentrates. Transfus Med Hemother 2011; 38:33–42.

22. North A, Ciaravino V, Mufti N, et al. Preclinical pharmacokinetics and toxicology assessment of red blood cells prepared with S-303 pathogen inactivation treatment. Transfusion 2011;51:2208–18.

23. Cancelas JA, Gottschall JL, Rugg N, et al. Red blood cell concentrates treated with the amustaline (S-303) pathogen reduction system and stored for 35 days retain post-transfusion viability: results of a two-centre study. Transfusion 2017; 112:210–8.

24. Winter KM, Johnson L, Kwok M, et al. Red blood cell in vitro quality and function is maintained after S-303 pathogen inactivation treatment. Transfusion 2014;54: 1798–807.

25. Brixner V, Kiessling A-H, Madlener K, et al. Red blood cells treated with the amustaline (S-303) pathogen reduction system: a transfusion study in cardiac surgery. Transfusion 2018;58:905–16.
26. Mundt J, Rouse L, Van den Bossche J, et al. Chemical and biological mechanisms of pathogen reduction technologies. Photochem Photobiol 2014;90: 957–64.
27. Marschner S, Goodrich R. Pathogen reduction technology treatment of platelets, plasma and whole blood using riboflavin and UV light. Transfus Med Hemother 2011;38:8–18.
28. Fast LD, Dileon G, Li J, et al. Functional inactivation of white blood cells by Mirasol treatment. Transfusion 2006;46:642–8.
29. Jackman RP, Heitman JW, Marschner S, et al. Understanding loss of donor white blood cell immunogenicity following pathogen reduction: mechanisms of action in UV illumination and riboflavin treatment. Transfusion 2009;49:2686–99.
30. Jackman RP, Muench MO, Inglis H, et al. Reduced MHC alloimmunization and partial tolerance protection with pathogen reduction of whole blood. Transfusion 2017;57:337–48.
31. Tormey CA, Santhanakrishnan M, Smith NH, et al. Riboflavin-ultraviolet light pathogen reduction treatment does not impact the immunogenicity of murine red blood cells. Transfusion 2016;56:863–72.
32. TerumoBCT. Terumo BCT announces enrollment of the first patient in its U.S. clinical trial designed to study platelets treated with the Mirasol® pathogen reduction technology (PRT) system. [Press Release] 2017. Available at: https://www.terumobct.com/Pages/News/Press%20Releases/Terumo-BCT-Announces-Enrollment-of-the-First-Patient–in-Its-U-S–Clinical-Trial-Designed-to-Study-Platelets-Treated–With-.aspx. Accessed June 25, 2019.
33. Seltsam A, Muller TH. UVC irradiation for pathogen reduction of platelet concentrates and plasma. Transfus Med Hemother 2011;38:43–54.
34. Seghatchain J, Tolksdorf F. Characteristics of the THERAFLEX UV-platelets pathogen inactivation system- an update. Transfus Apher Sci 2012;46:221–9.
35. Gravemann U, Wiebke H, Muller TH, et al. Bacterial inactivation of platelet concentrates with the THERAFLEX UV-platelets pathogen inactivation system. Transfusion 2019;59:1324–32.
36. Wagner SJ, Getz TM. Is a platelet suntan the answer? Transfusion 2019;59: 1163–5.
37. Mohr H, Steil L, Gravemann U, et al. Blood components: a novel approach to pathogen reduction in platelet concentrates using short-wave ultraviolet light. Transfusion 2009;49:2612–24.
38. Sinha RP, Hader DP. UV-induced DNA damage and repair: a review. Photochem Photobiol Sci 2002;1:225–36.
39. Verhaar R, Dekkers DW, De Cuyper IM, et al. UV-C irradiation disrupts platelet surface disulfide bonds and activates the platelet integrin alphaII/beta3. Blood 2008;112:4935–9.
40. Lytle CD, Sagripanti JL. Predicted inactivation of viruses of relevance to biodefense by solar radiation. J Virol 2005;79:14244–52.
41. Henderson EE, Tudor G, Yang JY. Inactivation of the human immunodeficiency virus type 1 (HIV-1) by ultraviolet and X irradiation. Radiat Res 1992;131:169–76.
42. Castro E, Gonzalez LM, Rubio JM, et al. The efficacy of the ultraviolet C pathogen inactivation system in the reduction of Babesia divergens in pooled buffy coat platelets. Transfusion 2014;54:2207–16.

43. Gravemann U, Pohler P, Lambrecht B, et al. Inactivation of peripheral blood mononuclear cells by UVC light using the theraflex UV-platelet system. Transfus Med Hemother 2008;35:4.

44. Hart H, Reid K, Hart W. Inactivation of viruses during ultraviolet light treatment of human intravenous immunoglobulin and albumin. Vox Sang 1993;64:82–8.

45. Chin S, Williams B, Gottlieb P, et al. Virucidal short wavelength ultraviolet light treatment of plasma and factor VIII concentrate: protection of proteins by anti-oxidants. Blood 1995;86:4331–6.

46. Floyd RA, Schneider JE, Dittmer D. Methylene blue photo-inactivation of RNA viruses. Antiviral Res 2004;61:141–51.

47. Wainwright M. Methylene blue derivatives: suitable photoantimicrobials for blood product disinfection? Int J Antimicrob Agents 2000;16:381–94.

48. Noens L, Vilarino MD, Megalou A, et al. International, prospective haemovigilance study on methylene blue treated plasma. Vox Sang 2017;112:352–9.

49. Seghatchian J, Struff WG, Reichenberg S. Main properties of the THERAFLEX MB-plasma system for pathogen reduction. Transfus Med Hemother 2011;38: 55–64.

50. Nubret K, Delhoume M, Orsel I, et al. Anaphylactic shock to fresh-frozen plasma inactivated with methylene blue. Transfusion 2011;51:125–8.

51. Bost V, Odent-Malaure H, Chavarin P, et al. A regional haemovigilance retro-spective study of four types of therapeutic plasma in a ten-year survey period in France. Vox Sang 2013;104:337–41.

52. Octaplas, pooled plasma (human), solvent/detergent treated solution for intra-venous infusion [package insert]. Hoboken (NJ): Octapharma USA Inc.; 2015.

53. Niesser-Svae A, Bailey A, Gregori L, et al. Prion removal effect of a specific af-finity ligand introduced into the manufacturing process of the pharmaceutical quality solvent/detergent (S/D)-treated plasma OctaplasLG®. Vox Sang 2009; 97:226–33.

54. Lawrie A, Green L, Canciani MT, et al. The effect of prion reduction in solvent/detergent-treated plasma on haemostatic variables. Vox Sang 2010;99:232–8.

55. Hellstern P, Solheim BG. The use of solvent/detergent treatment in pathogen reduction of plasma. Transfus Med Hemother 2011;38:65–70.

56. Chou M-L, Wu Y-W, Su C-Y, et al. Impact of solvent/detergent treatment of plasma on transfusion-relevant bacteria. Vox Sang 2011;102:277–84.

57. Cicchetti A, Berrino A, Casini M, et al. Health technology assessment of path-ogen reduction technologies applied to plasma for clinical use. Blood Transfus 2016;14:287–386.

58. Yazer MH, Jackson B, Sperry ML, et al. Initial safety and feasibility of cold-stored uncrossmatched whole blood transfusion in civilian trauma patients. J Trauma Acute Care Surg 2016;81:21–6.

59. Ware AD, Jacquot C, Tobian AAR, et al. Pathogen reduction and blood transfu-sion safety in Africa: strengths, limitations and challenges of implementation in low-resource settings. Vox Sang 2018;113:3–12.

60. Cotton BA, Podbielski J, Camp E, et al. A randomized controlled pilot trial of modified whole blood versus component therapy in severely injured patients requiring large volume transfusions. Ann Surg 2013;258:527–33.

61. Spinella PC, Perkins JG, Grathwohl KW, et al. Warm fresh whole blood is inde-pendently associated with improved survival for patients with combat-related traumatic injuries. J Trauma 2009;66:S69–76.

62. Jobes DR, Sesok-Pizzini D, Friedman D. Reduced transfusion requirement with use of fresh whole blood in pediatric cardiac surgical procedures. Ann Thorac Surg 2015;99:1706–12.

63. Cap AP, Beckett A, Benov A, et al. Whole blood transfusion. Mil Med 2018;183: 44–51.

64. Spinella P, Cap A. Whole blood: back to the future. Curr Opin Hematol 2016;23: 536–42.

65. Prowse CV. Component pathogen inactivation: a critical review. Vox Sang 2013; 104:183–99.

66. Tonnetti I, Thorp AM, Reddy HL, et al. Evaluating pathogen reduction of Trypanosoma cruzi with riboflavin and ultraviolet light for whole blood. Transfusion 2012;52:409–16.

67. Tonnetti I, Thorp AM, Reddy HI, et al. Riboflavin and ultraviolet light reduce the infectivity of Babesia microti in whole blood. Transfusion 2013;53:860–7.

68. Tonnetti I, Thorp AM, Reddy HI, et al. Reduction of Leishmania donovani infectivity in whole blood using riboflavin and ultraviolet light. Transfusion 2015;55: 326–9.

69. El Chaar M, Atwal S, Freimanis GL, et al. Inactivation of plasmodium falciparum in whole blood by riboflavin plus irradiation. Transfusion 2013;53: 3174–83.

70. Yonemura S, Doane S, Keil S, et al. Improving the safety of whole blood-derived transfusion products with a riboflavin-based pathogen reduction technology. Blood Transfus 2017;15:357–64.

71. Allain JP, Owusu-Ofori AK, Assennato SM, et al. Effect of plasmodium inactivation in whole blood on the incidence of blood transfusion-transmitted malaria in endemic regions: the African investigation of the Mirasol system (AIMS) randomized controlled trial. Lancet 2016;387:1753–61.

72. Allain JP, Goodrich R. Pathogen reduction of whole blood: utility and feasibility. Transfus Med 2017;27:320–6.

73. Cancelas JA, Slichter SJ, Rugg N, et al. Red blood cells derived from whole blood treated with riboflavin and ultraviolet light maintain adequate survival in vivo after 21 days of storage. Transfusion 2017;57:1218–25.

74. Trakhtman P, Kumukova I, Starostin N, et al. The pathogen-reduced red blood cell suspension: single centre study of clinical safety and efficacy in children with oncological and haematological diseases. Vox Sang 2019; 114:223–31.

75. US Food and Drug Administration/Center for Biologics Evaluation and Research. Bacterial risk control strategies for blood collection establishments and transfusion services to enhance the safety and availability of platelets for transfusion: draft guidance for industry. Available at: https://www.fda.gov/media/123448/download. Accessed June 25, 2019.

76. US Food and Drug Administration/Center for Biologics Evaluation and Research, Marks P. FY 2018 report from the director 2019. Silver Spring (MD): US Government. Available at: https://www.fda.gov/vaccines-blood-biologics/fy-2018-report-director. Accessed May 1, 2019.

77. Estcourt LJ, Malouf R, Hopewell S, et al. Pathogen-reduced platelets for the prevention of bleeding. Cochrane Database Syst Rev 2017;7:1–132.

78. Garban F, Guyard A, Labussiere H, et al. Comparison of the hemostatic efficacy of pathogen-reduced platelets vs. untreated platelets in patients with thrombocytopenia and malignant hematologic diseases. JAMA Oncol 2018;4:468–75.

79. Karafin M, Fuller AK, Savage WJ, et al. The impact of apheresis platelet manipulation on corrected count increment. Transfusion 2012;52:1221–7.
80. Mirasol Clinical Evaluation Study Group. A randomized controlled clinical trial evaluating the performance and safety of platelets treated with MIRASOL pathogen reduction technology. Transfusion 2010;50:2362–75.
81. Rebulla P, Vaglio S, Beccaria F, et al. Clinical effectiveness of platelets in additive solution treated with two commercial pathogen-reduction technologies. Transfusion 2017;57:1171–83.
82. Efficacy of Mirasol-treated Apheresis Platelets in Patients with Hypoproliferative Thrombocytopenia (MIPLATE). Available at: https://clinicaltrials.gov/ct2/show/NCT02964325. Accessed June 25, 2019.
83. Gehrie EA. Atypical bacterial growth within units of platelets challenges transfusion medicine dogma. J Clin Microbiol 2018;56 [pii:e01363-18].
84. Lozano M, Cid J, Muller T. Plasma treated with methylene blue and light: clinical efficacy and safety profile. Transfus Med Rev 2013;27:235–40.
85. Osselaer JC, Debry C, Goffaux M, et al. Coagulation function in fresh-frozen plasma prepared with two photochemical treatment methods: methylene blue and amotosalen. Transfusion 2008;48:108–17.
86. Cardigan R, Philpot K, Cookson P, et al. Thrombin generation and clot formation in methylene blue-treated plasma and cryoprecipitate. Transfusion 2009;49:696–703.
87. Alvarez-Larran A, Del Rio J, Ramirez C, et al. Methylene blue-photoinactivated plasma vs. fresh-frozen plasma as replacement fluid for plasma exchange in thrombotic thrombocytopenic purpura. Vox Sang 2004;86:246–51.
88. Svae TE, Frenzel W, Heger A, et al. Quality differences between solvent/detergent plasmas and fresh frozen plasma. Transfus Med 2007;17:318–20.
89. Hellstern P. Solvent/detergent-treated plasma: composition, efficacy, safety. Curr Opin Hematol 2004;11:346–50.
90. Neisser-Svae A, Trawnicek L, Heger A, et al. Five-day stability of thawed plasma: solvent/detergent-treated plasma comparable with fresh-frozen plasma and plasma frozen within 24 hours. Transfusion 2016;56:404–9.
91. Haubelt H, Blome M, Kiessling AH, et al. Effects of solvent/detergent-treated plasma and fresh-frozen plasma on haemostasis and fibrinolysis in complex coagulopathy following open-heart surgery. Vox Sang 2002;82:9–14.
92. Watson JJ, Pati S, Schreiber MA. Plasma transfusion: history, current realities, and novel improvements. Shock 2016;46:468–79.
93. Octapharma. FDA approves Octaplas® expanding Octapharma US transfusion medicine therapies. [Press Release]. 2013. Available at: https://www.octapharma.com/en/about/newsroom/press-releases/news-single-view.html?tx_ttnews%5Btt_news%5D=404&cHash=886d2559eb3ac4e6f0a7526a35781cf7. Accessed June 25, 2019.
94. Solheim BG, Granov DA, Juravlev VA, et al. Universal fresh-frozen plasma (Uniplas): an exploratory study in adult patients undergoing elective liver resection. Vox Sang 2005;89:19–26.
95. Heger A, Brandstatter H, Prager B, et al. Universal pooled plasma (Uniplas®) does not induce complement-mediated hemolysis of the human red blood cells in vitro. Transfus Apher Sci 2015;52:128–35.
96. Cazenave JP, Waller C, Kientz D, et al. An active hemovigilance program characterizing the safety profile of 7483 transfusions with plasma components prepared with amotosalen and UVA photochemical treatment. Transfusion 2010;50:1210–9.

97. Mintz PD, Neff A, MacKenzie M, et al. A randomized, controlled Phase III trial of therapeutic plasma exchange with fresh-frozen plasma (FFP) prepared with amotosalen and ultraviolet A light compared to untreated FFP in thrombotic thrombocytopenic purpura. Transfusion 2006;46:1693–704.

98. Ciaravino V, McCullough T, Cimino G, et al. Preclinical safety profile of plasma prepared using the INTERCEPT Blood System. Vox Sang 2003;85:171–82.

99. Hawkins BM, Abu-Fadel M, Vesely SK, et al. Clinical cardiac involvement in thrombotic thrombocytopenic purpura: a systematic review. Transfusion 2008; 48:382–92.

100. Erickson A, Waldhaus K, David T, et al. Plasma treated with amotosalen and ultraviolet A light retains activity for hemostasis after 5 days post-thaw storage at 1 to 6 C. Transfusion 2017;57:997–1006.

101. De Valensart N, Rapaille A, Goossenaerts E, et al. Study of coagulation function in thawed apheresis plasma for photochemical treatment by amotosalen and UVA. Vox Sang 2009;3:213–8.

102. Hubbard T, Backholer L, Wiltshire M, et al. Effects of riboflavin and amotosalen photoactivation systems for pathogen inactivation of fresh frozen plasma on fibrin clot structure. Transfusion 2016;56:41–8.

103. Ramirez-Arcos S, Jenkins C, Sheffield WP. Bacteria can proliferate in thawed cryoprecipitate stored at room temperature for longer than 4h. Vox Sang 2017;112:477–9.

104. Circular of information for the use of human blood and blood components. Bethesda (MD): AABB; 2017. Available at: http://www.aabb.org/tm/coi/Documents/coi1017.pdf. Accessed February 14, 2019.

105. Cid J, Caballo C, Pino M, et al. Quantitative and qualitative analysis of coagulation factors in cryoprecipitate prepared from fresh-frozen plasma inactivated with amotosalen and ultraviolet A light. Transfusion 2013;53:600–5.

106. Backholer L, Wiltshire M, Proffitt S, et al. Paired comparison of methylene blue- and amotosalen-treated plasma and cryoprecipitate. Vox Sang 2016;110:352–61.

107. Ettinger A, Miklauz MM, Bihm DJ, et al. Preparation of cryoprecipitate from riboflavin and UV-light treated plasma. Transfus Apher Sci 2012;46:153–8.

108. Burnouf T, Goubran HA, Radosevich M, et al. A minipool process for solvent-detergent treatment of cryoprecipitate at blood centres using a disposable bag system. Vox Sang 2006;91:56–62.

109. Burnouf T, Radosevich M, El-Ekiaby M, et al. Pathogen reduction technique for fresh-frozen plasma, cryoprecipitate, and plasma fraction minipools prepared in disposable processing bag systems. Transfusion 2011;51:446–7.

110. Bloch EM, Marshall CE, Boyd JS, et al. Implementation of secondary bacterial culture testing of platelets to mitigate residual risk of septic transfusion reactions. Transfusion 2018;58:1647–53.

111. Laughhunn A, Huang YS, Vanlandingham DL, et al. Inactivation of chikungunya virus in blood components treated with amotosalen/ultraviolet A light or amustaline/glutathione. Transfusion 2018;58:748–57.

112. Hauser I, Roque-Afonso AM, Beyloune A, et al. Hepatitis E transmission by transfusion of Intercept blood system treated plasma. Blood 2014;123:796–7.

113. Alvarez M, Luis-Hidalgo M, Bracho MA, et al. Transmission of human immunodeficiency virus type-1 by fresh-frozen plasma treated with methylene blue and light. Transfusion 2016;56:831–6.

114. Stolla M. Pathogen reduction and HLA alloimmunization: more questions than answers. Transfusion 2019;59:1152–5.

115. Russell WA, Stramer SL, Busch MP, et al. Screening the blood supply for Zika virus in the 50 US states and Puerto Rico. Ann Intern Med 2019;170:164–74.
116. Ellingson KD, Kuehnert MJ. Blood safety and emerging infections: balancing risks and costs. Ann Intern Med 2019;170:203–4.
117. Rutter A, Snyder EL. How do we…integrate pathogen reduced platelets into our hospital blood bank inventory? Transfusion 2019;59(5):1628–36.

Transfusion-Associated Circulatory Overload and Transfusion-Related Acute Lung Injury: Etiology and Prevention

Nareg H. Roubinian, MD, MPHTM[a,b,c,*], Darrell J. Triulzi, MD[d,e]

KEYWORDS

• Etiology • Prevention • Pulmonary transfusion reactions

KEY POINTS

- Donor/component mitigation strategies and patient blood management have decreased the incidence of pulmonary transfusion reactions.
- Transfusion-related acute lung injury (TRALI) and transfusion-associated circulatory overload (TACO) remain difficult to identify and diagnose.
- Cytokines and biomarkers may have utility in differentiating TRALI from TACO and Possible TRALI.
- Clinical and laboratory investigations are increasingly focused on identifying at-risk individuals and preventing pulmonary transfusion reactions.

INTRODUCTION

Systematic data collection has advanced our understanding of the incidence and epidemiology of transfusion-related acute lung injury (TRALI) and transfusion-associated circulatory overload (TACO).[1–6] These frequently severe complications of transfusion account for the majority of transfusion-related deaths and have been independently associated with morbidity and mortality.[7–10] However, in the past decade, donor/component mitigation and patient blood management strategies have reduced the incidence of pulmonary transfusion reactions. This review summarizes their risk factors, pathophysiology, and the role for biomarkers in the identification and differentiation of TRALI, TACO, and Possible TRALI to aid in their further prevention.

Disclosures: N.H. Roubinian and D.J. Triulzi have no conflicts of interest to disclose.
[a] Division of Research, Kaiser Permanente Northern California, Oakland, CA, USA; [b] Vitalant Research Institute, San Francisco, CA, USA; [c] University of California, San Francisco, San Francisco, CA, USA; [d] University of Pittsburgh, 3636 Boulevard of the Allies, Pittsburgh, PA 15213, USA; [e] Institute for Transfusion Medicine, Pittsburgh, PA, USA
* Corresponding author. 270 Masonic Avenue, San Francisco, CA 94118.
E-mail address: Nareg.H.Roubinian@kp.org

Hematol Oncol Clin N Am 33 (2019) 767–779
https://doi.org/10.1016/j.hoc.2019.05.003
0889-8588/19/© 2019 Elsevier Inc. All rights reserved.

DEFINITIONS

Challenges in the recognition and classification of pulmonary transfusion reactions have long hindered their study.[11,12] Working groups have endeavored to refine the criteria for TRALI and TACO, recognizing that current definitions lacked specificity.[6,13–15] Common to pulmonary transfusion reactions is the development of acute pulmonary edema within 6 hours of blood transfusion, characterized by hypoxemia due to bilateral opacities on chest radiography. However, accurate diagnosis relies on interpretation of clinical, hemodynamic, and radiographic data that are resource intensive to extract and require expertise to interpret.[16] Therefore, many research studies of TACO and TRALI collect granular clinical data and use expert panels of clinicians with experience in both intensive care and transfusion medicine to review cases.[1,8,17]

TRALI is an immunologic reaction resulting in acute lung injury and occurs as a result of capillary leak in the absence of circulatory overload and other ongoing risk factors for acute respiratory distress syndrome (ARDS).[6,16] In contrast, Possible TRALI is defined as acute lung injury following transfusion but includes a clear temporal association with another ARDS risk factor such as sepsis or pneumonia. Lastly, TACO is acute hydrostatic pulmonary edema following transfusion, frequently in the setting of renal or cardiac impairment.[2] Consensus criteria for the diagnosis of TACO have been proposed, and supportive findings include concurrent systolic or diastolic dysfunction, elevated cardiac filling pressures by echocardiogram or heart catheterization, and increased B-type natriuretic peptide (BNP) levels.

INCIDENCE

The reported incidence of TACO and TRALI has varied significantly with the method of case ascertainment, the patient population, and component type. Historically, incidence calculations were based on passively reported data from national hemovigilance, an approach known to underestimate incidence.[11,18,19] In the past decade, studies of pulmonary transfusion reactions have used active surveillance using electronic health record (EHR) screening to provide better estimates of their incidence.[1,5,12,20] Published rates have also varied with the studied patient population, with higher incidence in patients with increased comorbidity as well as frequency and diversity of blood component exposure. For example, active surveillance case series have reported TRALI in 0.1% of all transfused patients but in up to 8% of surgical or intensive care populations.[4,21–23] Some of the variability is also related to the inclusion or exclusion of more frequent Possible TRALI cases in TRALI estimates of both hemovigilance and active surveillance surveys.[4,21,22,24] In parallel, case series of TACO have reported higher incidence related to plasma transfusion and in perioperative or critically ill populations (1% to 4% of transfused patients).[2,5,21,25] Lastly, changes in blood collection and transfusion practice have been associated with reductions in reported incidence rates of TACO and TRALI. Prospective studies of TRALI have found lower incidence (~0.001% of transfused patients) following implementation of donor mitigation strategies.[1,8] In parallel, recent studies conducted following the advent of patient blood management programs reported a lower incidence of TACO (~1% of all transfused patients) than previously reported.[2,3,5,8,12,25]

CLINICAL PRESENTATION AND RISK FACTORS

Signs and symptoms of pulmonary edema typically occur within 6 hours of initiation of blood transfusion and include tachycardia, tachypnea, and hypoxia. Symptoms and associated requirements for supplemental oxygen and ventilatory support can occur acutely and sometimes be quite severe. However, the clinical course of patients with Possible TRALI and ARDS often progressively worsens over several days, whereas cases of TACO or TRALI may be more self-limited and responsive to supportive measures.

The total number of transfused blood products is an independent risk factor for both TACO and TRALI regardless of component type.[1] Blood components with a high plasma volume (eg, whole blood, apheresis platelet concentrates, or plasma products) historically conferred the highest risk for TRALI. Plasma-rich donations from previously pregnant women are a well-established risk factor for TRALI, and a dose-response increase in the prevalence of antileukocyte antibodies has been correlated with donor parity.[1,26–29] For TACO, the association with plasma transfusion is likely related to the large volume of blood components used to reverse coagulopathy, frequently in patients with impaired cardiac and renal function.[3,5,8]

Cardiovascular risk factors are common in TACO; patients tend to be older and have hypertension, coronary artery disease, or a history of congestive heart failure (**Table 1**).[2,3] Chronic renal impairment, including need for hemodialysis, is a frequent risk factor in cases of TACO, whereas acute kidney disease is prevalent in both TRALI and Possible TRALI.[2,5,21,30] Both TACO and TRALI are associated with perioperative transfusion, whereby more than half of cases of each occurred following surgery in one series.[2,5,31] TRALI and Possible TRALI have also been independently associated with liver disease, although this risk factor has not been reevaluated following plasma mitigation.[1,30,32] Although hypertension has frequently been associated with TACO, hypotension occurs commonly as well, with approximately half of TACO, TRALI, and Possible TRALI cases requiring vasopressor support in one study.[31] A positive

Table 1
Characteristics of cases and transfused controls from Specialized Clinical Center for Outcomes Research on transfusion-related acute lung injury

	TRALI n = 89	Possible TRALI n = 130	TACO n = 83	Control n = 164
Comorbid characteristics				
History of congestive heart failure	7 (8%)	8 (6%)	29 (35%)	13 (8%)
Coronary artery disease	15 (17%)	31 (24%)	34 (41%)	30 (18%)
Acute renal failure	23 (26%)	34 (26%)	15 (18%)	17 (10%)
Chronic renal failure	5 (6%)	11 (12%)	15 (18%)	14 (9%)
Severe liver disease	21 (24%)	20 (15%)	9 (11%)	15 (9%)
Recent surgery	54 (61%)	49 (38%)	62 (75%)	68 (41%)
Clinical characteristics				
Shock before transfusion	39 (44%)	59 (45%)	32 (39%)	30 (18%)
Ventilation after transfusion	42 (47%)	68 (52%)	56 (67%)	39 (24%)
Reduced ejection fraction (n = 263)	2/51 (4%)	12/75 (16%)	20/75 (29%)	11/67 (16%)
Elevated central venous pressure (n = 254)	4/50 (8%)	35/97 (36%)	21/67 (31%)	6/40 (15%)

Subjects from the TRALI SCCOR (Specialized Clinical Center for Outcomes Research) study—2006 to 2009.[1]

Data are reported as number (%).

Adapted from Roubinian NH, Looney MR, Kor DJ, et al. Cytokines and clinical predictors in distinguishing pulmonary transfusion reactions. Transfusion 2015;55(8):1838–1846; with permission.

fluid balance, while recognized as an independent risk factor for all pulmonary transfusion reactions, does not seem to be useful in their differentiation (**Table 2**).

PATHOGENESIS
Transfusion-related Acute Lung Injury

TRALI is thought to be due to passive transfusion of either antibody or nonantibody biological response modifiers (BRM) in the plasma of blood components. In antibody-mediated TRALI, the demonstration of human leukocyte or neutrophil antibodies in blood donor plasma with specificities against cognate (ie, corresponding) recipient antigens provides evidence for this hypothesis.[1,18,33] This hypothesis is further supported by in vivo models in which TRALI develops after donor leukocytes are infused into animals expressing cognate antigens.[34,35] In approximately 25% of TRALI cases, human leukocyte antibodies are not identified despite the use of sensitive assays.[36,37] These cases of "nonantibody-mediated" TRALI are thought to be due to either unidentified antibodies or other inflammatory factors within the transfused blood component. Although animal models have supported a role for inflammatory cytokines, soluble CD40 ligand, and nonpolar lipids (lysophosphatidylcholines) associated with prolonged storage, nonantibody mediators have not been associated with TRALI in human case-control studies.[1,23,38]

With advances in our understanding of TRALI pathogenesis, it was recognized that only a minority of transfused blood products containing human leukocyte antigen (HLA) antibodies result in TRALI.[39] Murine models and human studies suggest that systemic inflammation in the transfusion recipient is critical to TRALI pathogenesis as part of a 2-event hypothesis. In vivo models showed that lipopolysaccharide or other inflammatory stimuli (first event) are required for HLA antigen/antibody interactions (second event) to induce lung injury.[35] In cases of human TRALI, inflammatory conditions, associated with pretransfusion elevations in inflammatory cytokines interleukin 6 (IL-6) and IL-8 as well as C-reactive protein (CRP), are thought to play an important role in neutrophil priming before TRALI induction.[31,40,41]

Possible Transfusion-related Acute Lung Injury

In parallel with TRALI, patients who develop Possible TRALI are frequently exposed to potent inflammatory stimuli such as sepsis or pneumonia before transfusion. In these cases, the role of transfusion in the development of lung injury in patients with ARDS risk factors continues to be debated.[42,43] Although pretransfusion elevations in inflammatory cytokines such as IL-8 are prominent, antileukocyte antibodies are infrequent in Possible TRALI.[26,30] In addition, a male-predominant plasma strategy failed to reduce the Possible TRALI incidence raising questions regarding the role of

Table 2
Fluid balance in transfusion-related acute lung injury, possible transfusion-related acute lung injury, and transfusion-associated circulatory overload

	TACO	TRALI	Possible TRALI	P-Value
Rana et al,[21] 2006	5.9 (2.0–7.2)	4.8 (1.6–7.7)[a]	—	.21
Li et al,[24] 2009	3.2 (1.0–5.0)	4.8 (1.9–10.0)	5.0 (0.8–8.5)	.02
Clifford et al,[54] 2013	1.4 (0.2–3.5)	2.0 (0.7–4.1)[a]	—	.21
Roubinian et al,[31] 2015	3.7 (1.6–6)	3.7 (1.6–7.3)	4.4 (1.5–7.2)	.59

Data are presented as median values in liters (interquartile range).
[a] Combination of TRALI and Possible TRALI cases.

transfusion in its pathogenesis.[1,17,30] Lastly, the clinical course of Possible TRALI has been shown to differ from that of TRALI.[30,32] Given similarities in the pathophysiology and outcomes of Possible TRALI and ARDS, a working group is reconsidering the nomenclature for Possible TRALI.[42] Cases with ARDS risk factors such as sepsis thought to be driving lung injury may be considered "transfused ARDS" or ARDS, whereas those with clinical stability before transfusion and temporal separation from these risk factors may represent a subtype of TRALI. Clarification of this nomenclature would be beneficial given confusion regarding adverse event reporting and donor deferral in cases with ARDS risk factors.

Transfusion-associated Circulatory Overload

In TACO, elevated hydrostatic pressure with transfusion results in increased fluid filtration into the alveolar space and the development of a protein-poor pulmonary edema fluid.[44] Blood transfusion increases pulmonary capillary pressures more significantly than an equivalent volume of intravenous crystalloid fluid, potentially accounting for its designation from other causes of volume overload.[45,46] Similar to other mechanisms of hydrostatic pulmonary edema, TACO frequently occurs in patients with cardiac or renal impairment who are unable to compensate for increases in circulating blood volumes.[2]

The differentiation of pulmonary transfusion reactions remains challenging; however, data on the role of brain natriuretic peptides (BNP), inflammatory cytokines, and echocardiography may serve to help with their distinction.

BRAIN NATRIURETIC PEPTIDES

BNP (and N-terminal pro-BNP) testing has played a major role in the differential diagnosis of cases of pulmonary edema, including those with TACO and TRALI.[47,48] In parallel with patients with congestive heart failure, BNP levels are elevated in cases of TACO.[49,50] In addition to circulatory overload, BNP may be elevated through other mechanisms, such as hypoxia or increased catecholamines.[51,52] Increased BNP levels have also been reported in ARDS and Possible TRALI in which nearly one-third of cases had elevated cardiac filling pressures consistent with concomitant hydrostatic edema.[24,51,53] Several studies found higher BNP levels in cases of TACO and Possible TRALI as compared with cases of TRALI.[24,48,54] In Possible TRALI, it may be that transfusion leads to elements of both hydrostatic and inflammatory pulmonary edema. It is important to recognize that the specificity of BNP levels may be decreased in patients with renal insufficiency, and sensitivity is reduced in patients with increased body mass index.[55,56] Nevertheless, BNP levels seem to have practical utility in differentiating TRALI from TACO and Possible TRALI (**Table 3**).[48]

INFLAMMATORY CYTOKINES

Clinical studies have found increased levels of the inflammatory cytokine IL-8 but lower levels of the antiinflammatory cytokine IL-10 in TRALI as compared with those of Possible TRALI.[1,31,57] These cytokines may be associated with a specific immune phenotype related to TRALI pathogenesis. Recently, regulatory T cells and dendritic cells were shown to be protective in murine models of antibody-mediated TRALI, and this protection was associated with increased levels of IL-10.[58,59] In addition, IL-10 administration prevented murine TRALI and reduced its severity following induction with anti-major histocompatibility complex class I antibodies. Additional studies are needed to confirm these findings in humans and further elaborate their role in TRALI pathogenesis.

Table 3
Natriuretic peptide levels before and following transfusion in transfusion-related acute lung injury, possible transfusion-related acute lung injury, and transfusion-associated circulatory overload

	TRALI	Possible TRALI	TACO	P-Value
Pre-Transfusion				
BNP (n = 23)[24]	170 (41–407)	85 (49–291)	521.5 (143–2180)	.13
BNP (n = 49)[48]	70 (16–278)	298 (101–786)	1091 (668–2030)	<.01
NT-proBNP (n = 61)[24]	664 (138–2402)	948 (232–2352)	3410 (686–11,952)	.02
Post-Transfusion				
BNP (n = 73)[24]	375 (122.5–781)	446 (128–743)	559 (288–1348)	.038
BNP (n = 68)[48]	271 (137–638)	686 (379–1431)	1934 (1552–3000)	<.01
NT-proBNP (n = 84)[24]	1559 (628–5114)	2349 (919–4610)	5197 (1695–15,714)	<.01

Natriuretic peptide levels are presented as median values in pg/mL (interquartile range).
Abbreviations: BNP, brain natriuretic peptide; NT-proBNP, N-terminal pro-brain natriuretic peptide.

The role for recipient inflammation in the pathogenesis of TACO remains an area of debate. Case series have found that a systemic inflammatory response including fevers occurs in some patients with TACO.[60] Studies have shown elevations in the inflammatory cytokine IL-8 before transfusion in patients who develop TRALI and Possible TRALI but not TACO.[1,31,32,41] These studies did not control for perioperative status and other comorbidities that may be associated with both a systematic inflammatory response and transfusion. In parallel to natriuretic peptides, a combination of inflammatory cytokines may be useful in differentiating TACO from TRALI and Possible TRALI following transfusion.[31]

ECHOCARDIOGRAPHY

Echocardiography provides a noninvasive assessment of cardiac function—information that can be beneficial in the differentiation of pulmonary transfusion reactions.[3,53,61] It has largely replaced invasive hemodynamic monitoring and frequently identifies abnormalities unrecognized clinically.[7,62] In the setting of pulmonary edema, echocardiographic findings of evidence of systolic and/or diastolic dysfunction or elevated cardiac filling pressures suggest circulatory overload.[3] Although common in TACO, cardiac dysfunction is also known to occur in Possible TRALI (see **Table 1**), supporting a hydrostatic in addition to inflammatory basis for pulmonary edema in these cases.[31] In contrast to TACO and Possible TRALI, the absence of echocardiographic abnormalities is central to the diagnosis of TRALI.

MITIGATION AND PREVENTION

Data from hemovigilance reporting mechanisms and active surveillance studies show that mitigation strategies have led to significant reductions in TRALI incidence.[63–67] Preferential distribution of male donor plasma, thus limiting exposure to donor leukocyte antibodies from previously pregnant female blood donors, resulted in declines in reported rates of TRALI.[1,64] In fact, following male-only plasma collection, the per component rate TRALI reported to the American Red Cross was higher in red blood cells and apheresis platelet compared with male-donor predominant plasma components.[68]

Following plasma mitigation, it was recognized that the rate of TRALI was approximately 6-fold higher from female as compared with male apheresis platelet donors. Concern that the platelet supply would not be able to support conversion to male-only donations led to a strategy to screen female apheresis platelet donors for leukocyte antibodies. An approach to distribute apheresis platelets exclusively collected from men, women who have never been pregnant, or women with negative HLA antibody test results following their most recent pregnancy further reduced TRALI incidence in combination with other measures.[69,70]

In one study, the residual risk of TRALI from plasma transfusion was predominantly due to group AB female donors—universally compatible plasma donors in short supply yet high demand.[71] Although most of the group AB plasma components were from male donors, 40% were from female donors unscreened for HLA antibodies and therefore with an associated increased risk for TRALI. Component modifications may serve as a practical approach to reducing the residual risk of TRALI from these types of blood products. Additive solutions and pooling of platelet and plasma components from multiple donors may dilute or neutralize HLA or human neutrophil antigen leukocyte antibodies.[72] For example, solvent/detergent plasma products derived from pooled human plasma result in lower antibody titers and/or antibody neutralization and seem to reduce TRALI incidence.[65,73,74]

Ongoing clinical research may also serve to improve the safety of transfusion practice and further prevent TACO and TRALI. Recent findings supported the safety of group A plasma in trauma situations rather than universally ABO-compatible group AB plasma.[75] Additional data on the use of alternatives to AB plasma may further reduce the need for collection of higher-risk female plasma due to blood supply limitations and thus the risk of TRALI. Hemostatic agents, such as factor concentrates or antifibrinolytics, are being increasingly used as alternatives to emergency plasma transfusion; a small clinical trial of patients requiring reversal of anticoagulation found that 4-factor prothrombin complex concentrate was associated with a reduced incidence of pulmonary edema compared with plasma.[76]

Widespread adoption of patient blood management (PBM) has also played a role in reducing the incidence of pulmonary transfusion reactions. The number of blood components transfused is a risk factor for pulmonary transfusion reactions, and restrictive transfusion practice is a core tenet of PBM. A meta-analysis of clinical trial data showed that a restrictive compared with liberal transfusion strategy was associated with a lower frequency of pulmonary edema.[77] Globally, patient blood management strategies have led to substantial declines in blood transfusion, and recent active surveillance studies reported lower incidence of TACO and TRALI than prior surveys.[78–82]

FUTURE DIRECTIONS

Future strategies for the prevention of TRALI focus on the identification of individuals at increased risk of adverse transfusion reactions. TRALI is known to occur in a minority of patients exposed to blood products from previously implicated donors. Studies suggest that a distinct immune phenotype may be present in patients who develop TRALI compared with other forms of lung injury.[58,59] Proposed immune-based strategies to prevent or treat TRALI include the targeting of CRP, IL-8, IL-10, reactive oxidative species, neutrophil extracellular traps, or Fc receptors of the recipient.[83] However, additional studies are needed to confirm that human pathophysiology parallels the results of murine models before embarking on clinical trials of TRALI.

In contrast to TRALI, few in vivo investigations have been conducted to further understand the pathogenesis of TACO. Recently, a rat model of TACO has been developed to better assess the effect of blood transfusion relative to other intravenous fluids on pulmonary capillary pressures, specific rates of blood administration, as well as the benefit of prophylactic diuretics on TACO incidence.[7,84] This model could also serve to study the role of systemic inflammation and BRM, such as free hemoglobin or nitric oxide scavengers, which have been hypothesized to contribute to TACO pathogenesis.[85–87]

Translating results of laboratory and human investigations of TACO and TRALI into clinical practice requires better identification and differentiation of at-risk individuals. Although clinical research studies have used EHR, implementation science research is needed to better harness its ever-expanding role in health care delivery. Currently, the Food and Drug Administration is leading an effort to apply natural language processing and machine-learning methods to EHR data to allow for more widespread surveillance of adverse events, including pulmonary transfusion reactions. Automated identification and reporting of transfusion reactions using blood donor, component, and recipient data could also allow assessment of the safety of modifications to blood components (eg, pathogen-reduced products or extended storage of platelets).

As predictive algorithms of adequate sensitivity and specificity are developed and embedded within the EHR, patients at increased risk of an adverse pulmonary transfusion event could be identified before transfusion.[12,54] Current research focuses on the use of biomarker screening and recursive partitioning algorithms to identify the patients at highest risk for TACO.[88] Identification of high-risk individuals could be coupled with clinical trial or practice interventions. For example, clinical decision support systems incorporating blood pressure measurements or creatinine clearance could trigger an alert to clinicians with recommendations for diuretic administration or alternatives to transfusion for individuals at increased risk for TACO. The continued collaboration of bench and clinical researchers to incorporate cytokine and biomarker phenotyping into predictive algorithms could advance the prevention and treatment of these frequently severe complications of blood transfusion.

ACKNOWLEDGMENTS

The authors wish to thank Drs Evan Bloch and Elizabeth St. Lezin for their feedback and input on the review article.

REFERENCES

1. Toy P, Gajic O, Bacchetti P, et al. Transfusion-related acute lung injury: incidence and risk factors. Blood 2012;119(7):1757–67.
2. Murphy EL, Kwaan N, Looney MR, et al. Risk factors and outcomes in transfusion-associated circulatory overload. Am J Med 2013;126(4):357.e29-38.
3. Li G, Rachmale S, Kojicic M, et al. Incidence and transfusion risk factors for transfusion-associated circulatory overload among medical intensive care unit patients. Transfusion 2011;51(2):338–43.
4. Gajic O, Rana R, Winters JL, et al. Transfusion-related acute lung injury in the critically ill: prospective nested case-control study. Am J Respir Crit Care Med 2007; 176(9):886–91.
5. Clifford L, Jia Q, Yadav H, et al. Characterizing the epidemiology of perioperative transfusion-associated circulatory overload. Anesthesiology 2015;122(1):21–8.
6. Kleinman S, Caulfield T, Chan P, et al. Toward an understanding of transfusion-related acute lung injury: statement of a consensus panel. Transfusion 2004; 44(12):1774–89.

7. Clifford L, Jia Q, Subramanian A, et al. Risk factors and clinical outcomes associated with perioperative transfusion-associated circulatory overload. Anesthesiology 2017;126(3):409–18.

8. Roubinian NH, Hendrickson JE, Triulzi DJ, et al. Contemporary risk factors and outcomes of transfusion-associated circulatory overload. Crit Care Med 2018; 46(4):577–85.

9. Bolton-Maggs PHB. Serious hazards of transfusion - conference report: celebration of 20 years of UK haemovigilance. Transfus Med 2017;27(6):393–400.

10. Fatalities reported to FDA following blood collection and transfusion 2016. Available at: https://www.fda.gov/downloads/BiologicsBloodVaccines/Safety Availability/ReportaProblem/TransfusionDonationFatalities/UCM598243.pdf. Accessed January 23, 2019.

11. Hendrickson JE, Roubinian NH, Chowdhury D, et al. Incidence of transfusion reactions: a multicenter study utilizing systematic active surveillance and expert adjudication. Transfusion 2016;56(10):2587–96.

12. Roubinian NH, Hendrickson JE, Triulzi DJ, et al. Incidence and clinical characteristics of transfusion-associated circulatory overload using an active surveillance algorithm. Vox Sang 2017;112(1):56–63.

13. Goldman M, Webert KE, Arnold DM, et al. Proceedings of a consensus conference: towards an understanding of TRALI. Transfus Med Rev 2005;19(1):2–31.

14. Goldman M, Land K, Robillard P, et al. Development of standard definitions for surveillance of complications related to blood donation. Vox Sang 2016;110(2): 185–8.

15. AuBuchon JP, Fung M, Whitaker B, et al. AABB validation study of the CDC's National Healthcare Safety Network Hemovigilance Module adverse events definitions protocol. Transfusion 2014;54(8):2077–83.

16. Gajic O, Gropper MA, Hubmayr RD. Pulmonary edema after transfusion: how to differentiate transfusion-associated circulatory overload from transfusion-related acute lung injury. Crit Care Med 2006;34(5 Suppl):S109–13.

17. Clifford L, Jia Q, Subramanian A, et al. Characterizing the epidemiology of postoperative transfusion-related acute lung injury. Anesthesiology 2015;122(1): 12–20.

18. Kopko PM, Marshall CS, MacKenzie MR, et al. Transfusion-related acute lung injury: report of a clinical look-back investigation. JAMA 2002;287(15):1968–71.

19. Hendrickson JE, Hillyer CD. Noninfectious serious hazards of transfusion. Anesth Analg 2009;108(3):759–69.

20. Finlay HE, Cassorla L, Feiner J, et al. Designing and testing a computer-based screening system for transfusion-related acute lung injury. Am J Clin Pathol 2005;124(4):601–9.

21. Rana R, Fernández-Pérez ER, Khan SA, et al. Transfusion-related acute lung injury and pulmonary edema in critically ill patients: a retrospective study. Transfusion 2006;46(9):1478–83.

22. Vlaar AP, Binnekade JM, Prins D, et al. Risk factors and outcome of transfusion-related acute lung injury in the critically ill: a nested case-control study. Crit Care Med 2010;38(3):771–8.

23. Vlaar AP, Hofstra JJ, Determann RM, et al. The incidence, risk factors, and outcome of transfusion-related acute lung injury in a cohort of cardiac surgery patients: a prospective nested case-control study. Blood 2011;117(16):4218–25.

24. Li G, Daniels CE, Kojicic M, et al. The accuracy of natriuretic peptides (brain natriuretic peptide and N-terminal pro-brain natriuretic) in the differentiation between

transfusion-related acute lung injury and transfusion-related circulatory overload in the critically ill. Transfusion 2009;49(1):13–20.

25. Narick C, Triulzi DJ, Yazer MH. Transfusion-associated circulatory overload after plasma transfusion. Transfusion 2012;52(1):160–5.

26. van Stein D, Beckers EA, Sintnicolaas K, et al. Transfusion-related acute lung injury reports in the Netherlands: an observational study. Transfusion 2010; 50(1):213–20.

27. Eder AF, Herron R, Strupp A, et al. Transfusion-related acute lung injury surveillance (2003-2005) and the potential impact of the selective use of plasma from male donors in the American Red Cross. Transfusion 2007;47(4):599–607.

28. Gajic O, Yilmaz M, Iscimen R, et al. Transfusion from male-only versus female donors in critically ill recipients of high plasma volume components. Crit Care Med 2007;35(7):1645–8.

29. Triulzi DJ, Kleinman S, Kakaiya RM, et al. The effect of previous pregnancy and transfusion on HLA alloimmunization in blood donors: implications for a transfusion-related acute lung injury risk reduction strategy. Transfusion 2009; 49(9):1825–35.

30. Toy P, Bacchetti P, Grimes B, et al. Recipient clinical risk factors predominate in possible transfusion-related acute lung injury. Transfusion 2015;55(5):947–52.

31. Roubinian NH, Looney MR, Kor DJ, et al. Cytokines and clinical predictors in distinguishing pulmonary transfusion reactions. Transfusion 2015;55(8):1838–46.

32. Looney MR, Roubinian N, Gajic O, et al. Prospective study on the clinical course and outcomes in transfusion-related acute lung injury*. Crit Care Med 2014;42(7): 1676–87.

33. Kopko PM, Popovsky MA, MacKenzie MR, et al. HLA class II antibodies in transfusion-related acute lung injury. Transfusion 2001;41(10):1244–8.

34. Silliman CC, Curtis BR, Kopko PM, et al. Donor antibodies to HNA-3a implicated in TRALI reactions prime neutrophils and cause PMN-mediated damage to human pulmonary microvascular endothelial cells in a two-event in vitro model. Blood 2007;109(4):1752–5.

35. Looney MR, Matthay MA. Animal models of transfusion-related acute lung injury. Crit Care Med 2006;34(5 Suppl):S132–6.

36. Middelburg RA, van Stein D, Briët E, et al. The role of donor antibodies in the pathogenesis of transfusion-related acute lung injury: a systematic review. Transfusion 2008;48(10):2167–76.

37. van Stein D, Beckers EA, Peters AL, et al. Underdiagnosing of antibody-mediated transfusion-related acute lung injury: evaluation of cellular-based versus bead-based techniques. Vox Sang 2016;111(1):71–8.

38. Tuinman PR, Gerards MC, Jongsma G, et al. Lack of evidence of CD40 ligand involvement in transfusion-related acute lung injury. Clin Exp Immunol 2011; 165(2):278–84.

39. Kleinman SH, Triulzi DJ, Murphy EL, et al. The Leukocyte Antibody Prevalence Study-II (LAPS-II): a retrospective cohort study of transfusion-related acute lung injury in recipients of high-plasma-volume human leukocyte antigen antibody-positive or -negative components. Transfusion 2011;51(10):2078–91.

40. Kapur R, Kim M, Rondina MT, et al. Elevation of C-reactive protein levels in patients with transfusion-related acute lung injury. Oncotarget 2016;7(47):78048–54.

41. Vlaar AP, Hofstra JJ, Determann RM, et al. Transfusion-related acute lung injury in cardiac surgery patients is characterized by pulmonary inflammation and coagulopathy: a prospective nested case-control study. Crit Care Med 2012;40(10): 2813–20.

42. Toy P, Kleinman SH, Looney MR. Proposed revised nomenclature for transfusion-related acute lung injury. Transfusion 2017;57(3):709–13.

43. Juffermans NP, Vlaar AP. Possible TRALI is a real entity. Transfusion 2017;57(10): 2539–41.

44. Ware LB, Matthay MA. Clinical practice. Acute pulmonary edema. N Engl J Med 2005;353(26):2788–96.

45. Gupta SP, Nand N, Gupta MS. Left ventricular filling pressures after rapid blood transfusion in cases of chronic severe anemia. Angiology 1982;33(5):343–8.

46. Nand N, Gupta MS, Sharma M. Effect of different amounts of blood transfusion given at different speeds on left ventricular filling pressure in cases of chronic severe anemia. Angiology 1986;37(4):281–4.

47. Maisel AS, Krishnaswamy P, Nowak RM, et al. Rapid measurement of B-type natriuretic peptide in the emergency diagnosis of heart failure. N Engl J Med 2002;347(3):161–7.

48. Roubinian NH, Looney MR, Keating S, et al. Differentiating pulmonary transfusion reactions using recipient and transfusion factors. Transfusion 2017;57(7): 1684–90.

49. Zhou L, Giacherio D, Cooling L, et al. Use of B-natriuretic peptide as a diagnostic marker in the differential diagnosis of transfusion-associated circulatory overload. Transfusion 2005;45(7):1056–63.

50. Tobian AA, Sokoll LJ, Tisch DJ, et al. N-terminal pro-brain natriuretic peptide is a useful diagnostic marker for transfusion-associated circulatory overload. Transfusion 2008;48(6):1143–50.

51. Semler MW, Marney AM, Rice TW, et al. B-Type natriuretic peptide, aldosterone, and fluid management in ARDS. Chest 2016;150(1):102–11.

52. Rivers EP, McCord J, Otero R, et al. Clinical utility of B-type natriuretic peptide in early severe sepsis and septic shock. J Intensive Care Med 2007;22(6):363–73.

53. Wheeler AP, Bernard GR, Thompson BT, et al. Pulmonary-artery versus central venous catheter to guide treatment of acute lung injury. N Engl J Med 2006; 354(21):2213–24.

54. Clifford L, Singh A, Wilson GA, et al. Electronic health record surveillance algorithms facilitate the detection of transfusion-related pulmonary complications. Transfusion 2013;53(6):1205–16.

55. Vickery S, Price CP, John RI, et al. B-type natriuretic peptide (BNP) and amino-terminal proBNP in patients with CKD: relationship to renal function and left ventricular hypertrophy. Am J Kidney Dis 2005;46(4):610–20.

56. Das SR, Drazner MH, Dries DL, et al. Impact of body mass and body composition on circulating levels of natriuretic peptides: results from the Dallas Heart Study. Circulation 2005;112(14):2163–8.

57. Kapur R, Kim M, Rebetz J, et al. Low levels of interleukin-10 in patients with transfusion-related acute lung injury. Ann Transl Med 2017;5(16):339.

58. Kapur R, Kim M, Aslam R, et al. T regulatory cells and dendritic cells protect against transfusion-related acute lung injury via IL-10. Blood 2017;129(18): 2557–69.

59. He R, Li L, Kong Y, et al. Preventing murine transfusion-related acute lung injury by expansion of $CD4^+$ $CD25^+$ $FoxP3^+$ Tregs using IL-2/anti-IL-2 complexes. Transfusion 2019;59(2):534–44.

60. Parmar N, Pendergrast J, Lieberman L, et al. The association of fever with transfusion-associated circulatory overload. Vox Sang 2017;112(1):70–8.

61. Lieberman L, Maskens C, Cserti-Gazdewich C, et al. A retrospective review of patient factors, transfusion practices, and outcomes in patients with

transfusion-associated circulatory overload. Transfus Med Rev 2013;27(4):
206–12.

62. Gaasch WH. Diagnosis and treatment of heart failure based on left ventricular systolic or diastolic dysfunction. JAMA 1994;271(16):1276–80.

63. Chapman CE, Stainsby D, Jones H, et al. Ten years of hemovigilance reports of transfusion-related acute lung injury in the United Kingdom and the impact of preferential use of male donor plasma. Transfusion 2009;49(3):440–52.

64. Eder AF, Herron RM, Strupp A, et al. Effective reduction of transfusion-related acute lung injury risk with male-predominant plasma strategy in the American Red Cross (2006-2008). Transfusion 2010;50(8):1732–42.

65. Ozier Y, Muller JY, Mertes PM, et al. Transfusion-related acute lung injury: reports to the French Hemovigilance Network 2007 through 2008. Transfusion 2011; 51(10):2102–10.

66. Jutzi M, Levy G, Taleghani BM. Swiss Haemovigilance data and implementation of measures for the prevention of transfusion associated acute lung Injury (TRALI). Transfus Med Hemother 2008;35(2):98–101.

67. Lin Y, Saw CL, Hannach B, et al. Transfusion-related acute lung injury prevention measures and their impact at Canadian Blood Services. Transfusion 2012;52(3): 567–74.

68. Eder AF, Dy BA, O'Neill EM. Predicted effect of selectively testing female donors for HLA antibodies to mitigate transfusion-related acute lung injury risk from apheresis platelets. Transfusion 2016;56(6 Pt 2):1608–15.

69. Lucas G, Win N, Calvert A, et al. Reducing the incidence of TRALI in the UK: the results of screening for donor leucocyte antibodies and the development of national guidelines. Vox Sang 2012;103(1):10–7.

70. Shaz BH. Bye-bye TRALI: by understanding and innovation. Blood 2014;123(22): 3374–6.

71. Eder AF, Dy BA, Perez JM, et al. The residual risk of transfusion-related acute lung injury at the American Red Cross (2008-2011): limitations of a predominantly male-donor plasma mitigation strategy. Transfusion 2013;53(7):1442–9.

72. Andreu G, Boudjedir K, Muller JY, et al. Analysis of transfusion-related acute lung injury and possible transfusion-related acute lung injury reported to the French Hemovigilance Network from 2007 to 2013. Transfus Med Rev 2018;32(1):16–27.

73. Sachs UJ, Kauschat D, Bein G. White blood cell-reactive antibodies are undetectable in solvent/detergent plasma. Transfusion 2005;45(10):1628–31.

74. Riedler GF, Haycox AR, Duggan AK, et al. Cost-effectiveness of solvent/detergent-treated fresh-frozen plasma. Vox Sang 2003;85(2):88–95.

75. Dunbar NM, Yazer MH, Biomedical Excellence for Safer Transfusion (BEST) Collaborative and the STAT Study Investigators. Safety of the use of group A plasma in trauma: the STAT study. Transfusion 2017;57(8):1879–84.

76. Sarode R, Milling TJ, Refaai MA, et al. Efficacy and safety of a 4-factor prothrombin complex concentrate in patients on vitamin K antagonists presenting with major bleeding: a randomized, plasma-controlled, phase IIIb study. Circulation 2013;128(11):1234–43.

77. Salpeter SR, Buckley JS, Chatterjee S. Impact of more restrictive blood transfusion strategies on clinical outcomes: a meta-analysis and systematic review. Am J Med 2014;127(2):124–31.e3.

78. Roubinian NH, Escobar GJ, Liu V, et al. Decreased red blood cell use and mortality in hospitalized patients. JAMA Intern Med 2014;174(8):1405–7.

79. Mazzeffi MA, See JM, Williams B, et al. Five-year trends in perioperative red blood cell transfusion from index cases in five surgical specialties: 2011 to 2015. Transfusion 2018;58(5):1271–8.

80. Ellingson KD, Sapiano MRP, Haass KA, et al. Continued decline in blood collection and transfusion in the United States-2015. Transfusion 2017;57(Suppl 2): 1588–98.

81. Freedman J. The ONTraC Ontario program in blood conservation. Transfus Apher Sci 2014;50(1):32–6.

82. Meybohm P, Herrmann E, Steinbicker AU, et al. Patient blood management is associated with a substantial reduction of red blood cell utilization and safe for patient's outcome: a prospective, multicenter cohort study with a noninferiority design. Ann Surg 2016;264(2):203–11.

83. Semple JW, McVey MJ, Kim M, et al. Targeting transfusion-related acute lung injury: the journey from basic science to novel therapies. Crit Care Med 2018; 46(5):e452–8.

84. Roubinian N, Murphy EL. Adjusting the focus on transfusion-associated circulatory overload. Anesthesiology 2017;126(3):363–5.

85. Warner MA, Welsby IJ, Norris PJ, et al. Point-of-care washing of allogeneic red blood cells for the prevention of transfusion-related respiratory complications (WAR-PRC): a protocol for a multicenter randomised clinical trial in patients undergoing cardiac surgery. BMJ Open 2017;7(8):e016398.

86. Donadee C, Raat NJ, Kanias T, et al. Nitric oxide scavenging by red blood cell microparticles and cell-free hemoglobin as a mechanism for the red cell storage lesion. Circulation 2011;124(4):465–76.

87. Risbano MG, Kanias T, Triulzi D, et al. Effects of aged stored autologous red blood cells on human endothelial function. Am J Respir Crit Care Med 2015; 192(10):1223–33.

88. Callum JL, Cohen R, Cressman AM, et al. Cardiac stress biomarkers after red blood cell transfusion in patients at risk for transfusion-associated circulatory overload: a prospective observational study. Transfusion 2018;58(9):2139–48.

Iron Depletion in Adult and Teenage Blood Donors

Prevalence, Clinical Impact, and Options for Mitigation

Bryan R. Spencer, PhD

KEYWORDS

- Iron • Iron depletion • Young blood donors

KEY POINTS

- Iron depletion is a well-known risk for adult blood donors; recent studies indicate the risk is higher in donors 16 to 18 years old.
- Evidence for severe clinical sequalae from donation-induced iron depletion is lacking, and in nondonor populations symptoms are more strongly associated with iron deficiency anemia.
- Some blood collectors have implemented interventions on a precautionary basis to protect against iron depletion in teen donors given their ongoing neurocognitive development.
- Potentially effective options to mitigate iron depletion exist, but each has substantive challenges relating to logistics, cost, and reduced availability of blood products.

INTRODUCTION

Despite a 30% decrease in blood collections since 2008, transfusion of blood products remains one of the most common medical procedures performed in the United States each year. Current reports indicate that approximately 11.3 million red cells, 2.9 million units of platelets, and 2.7 million units of plasma were transfused in 2015.[1] More than 10% of red cell units in recent years came from high school-age donors (16–18 years old).[2] Recent scientific inquiries into the prevalence and determinants of iron depletion (ID) in adult blood donors have cast a spotlight on the young donor population. Regulators, accreditors, and blood collectors are collectively assessing evidence for adverse consequences in teen donors, and whether additional protective measures might be indicated.

Disclosure: Dr B.R. Spencer is on the advisory board of HemaStrat, LLC.
Scientific Affairs, American Red Cross, 180 Rustcraft Road, Dedham, MA 02026, USA
E-mail address: bryan.spencer@redcross.org

Hematol Oncol Clin N Am 33 (2019) 781–796
https://doi.org/10.1016/j.hoc.2019.05.004
0889-8588/19/© 2019 Elsevier Inc. All rights reserved.

hemonc.theclinics.com

PREVALENCE OF AND RISK FACTORS FOR IRON DEFICIENCY IN BLOOD DONORS
Studies on Adult Donors in the United States

The potential for blood donation to contribute to iron deficiency has been known for decades. Finch and colleagues[3] showed that males averaging 3 donations per year had average ferritin values one-half that of those with 1 annual donation (approximately 31 ng/mL vs 70 ng/mL) and were more likely to have a ferritin of less than 12 ng/mL (12.7% vs 0.9%). They recorded a similar pattern in females, with the prevalence of a ferritin of less than 12 ng/mL reaching 26.8% in the females averaging 3 units per year. Simon and colleagues[4] recorded prevalence of a ferritin of less than 12 ng/mL in unselected donors of 8% in males and 23% in females, showing also that hemoglobin correlated poorly with iron stores. They also demonstrated that menstruation added to risk in females and even occasional iron supplementation improved iron stores. Studies in other countries[5] confirmed the findings of Simon and associates[4] that lifetime donations are less predictive of blood donor iron status than recent donation frequency. These results underscored that for many donors iron absorption failed to allow for return to equilibrium iron status under allowable inter-donation intervals.

In the absence of point-of-care assessment of iron status, blood centers have long relied on hemoglobin measurement as an indirect proxy for iron status. A 2001 industry workshop focused on the health of female donors of reproductive age, the importance of maintaining adequate iron status, and the adequacy of blood supply.[6] Presentations noted that premenopausal women account for 95% of 700,000 annual deferrals for low hemoglobin, permanent donor loss often follows deferral, and iron supplementation programs could improve the status quo. Although blood center implementation of iron supplementation protocols was constrained by an array of factors, studies in the United States and other countries have clarified the relationship between blood donation and ID and quantified the associations for many risk factors.

The REDS-II RISE study (**Table 1**) was a prospective cohort study seeking to characterize ID in a blood donor population and to identify and quantify risk factors. RISE investigators defined a ferritin of less than 12 ng/mL as absent iron stores (AIS), reflecting the level below which stainable iron is absent from the bone marrow. Values of the log ratio of soluble transferrin receptor/ferritin of 2.07 or greater was defined as iron-deficient erythropoiesis (IDE) to represent intermediate iron deficiency. At enrollment, the prevalence of AIS was 15% and of IDE was 41% across all 2425 participants. The range varied from 0% for AIS in first-time male donors to 66% IDE in the frequent female cohort (2 units of red blood cells donated per year).[7] In a longitudinal analysis, the RISE investigators helped to refine our understanding of blood donation and donor health, showing:

- Many of the demographic, behavioral, and donation-related risk factors evaluated differed in significance and magnitude between models predicting hemoglobin deferral and those for ID.
- Donation-related factors—frequency of donation and the interval since one's last donation—contributed the greatest predictive strength for blood donor iron status, and known genetic polymorphisms for iron homeostasis had modest associations with iron outcomes.
- The risk for AIS, a ferritin of less than 12 ng/mL, might last up to 5 months after a donation.

The latter point was especially notable. First, the outcome of AIS was not uncommon, documented in 22% of donor visits tested and estimated by a simulation study

Table 1
Selected studies on the prevalence and determinants of ID in blood donors

Study	Study Population & Design	Key Findings
RISE[7–9] (United States)	2425 first-time/reactivated[a] and frequent[b] adult donors; prospective cohort	50%–60% of frequent donors have intermediate or advanced ID Risk for AIS lasts 4–5 mo after donating Simulations indicate 13% of donors have AIS and 34% ferritin <26 ng/mL
STRIDE[10] (United States)	692 frequent[b] adult donors not taking iron; RCT with randomization to iron pills or educational treatments	Low-dose iron (19 mg) improves recovery of ferritin and hemoglobin and blood collections equivalent to 38 mg iron with negligible side effects Donors informed of their low ferritin values took recommended actions of delaying next donation or taking supplemental iron
HEIRS[11] (United States)	215 adult donors with no donation in 4 mo; RCT with randomization to 38 mg iron pills or no treatment	Without iron supplementation, two-thirds of donors do not recover hemoglobin or ferritin within 24 wk of donating With daily iron supplementation, average time to recovery of hemoglobin was 1 mo and to recovery of ferritin was 3–10 wk for those with initial ferritin values of ≤26 or >26 ng/mL, respectively
CHILL[12] (United States)	4265 donors, 16- to 18-year-olds and 19- to 49-year-old controls; prospective cohort	Donors 16–18 were 2 to 4 times more likely to have a ferritin of <12 or <26 ng/mL, respectively than 19- to 49-year-olds Hemoglobin deferral was twice as likely in 16-year-old girls compared with 19- to 49-year-old females, with low ferritin a major risk factor
Patel[13] (United States)	9647 adolescent and adult females age 16–49 y; representative cross-sectional sample	Prevalence of AIS was 23% in 16- to 19-year-old and 18% in 20–49-year-old females who donated within the last 12 mo Donation within last 12 mo was associated with approximately double the risk for AIS and for IDA for 16-to 19- and 20–49 year-olds
Canada[14,15]	12,595 donors ≥17-year-old; representative cross-sectional sample	Prevalence of ferritin <12 ng/mL was 17% and <25 ng/mL was 42% Notification of ferritin <25 ng/mL lead to 2-y donation decrease from 7.5 to 4.5 red cell units in male donors and from 5 to 3 units in females

(continued on next page)

Table 1 *(continued)*		
Study	**Study Population & Design**	**Key Findings**
Australia[16]	3049 donors age 16 and older; representative cross-sectional sample	Prevalence of ferritin <15 ng/mL was 13.6% and anemia was 4.2%. Predictive models showed poor sensitivity for ID
Netherlands[17]	5280 adult whole blood donors; cross-sectional sample	Prevalence of ID varied approximately 5-fold by assay in comparison study, from roughly 5%–25% in male and female donors

Abbreviations: AIS, absent iron stores (ferritin <12 ng/mL); IDA, iron deficiency anemia; RCT, randomized clinical trial.

[a] Reactivated donors were repeat donors, but had not donated within 2 years.

[b] Frequent donors had donated at least 2 red cell units in the year prior to enrollment if female, 3 if male.

to be prevalent in 13% of the overall donor population.[9] Second, the duration of risk for AIS after donation iron was considerably longer than the statutory minimum 8-week interval between donations in the United States.

Documentation of the sizable prevalence of ID motivated projects to evaluate mitigation strategies. The STRIDE study (see **Table 1**) enrolled frequent donors not using supplemental iron to identify the minimal efficacious intervention for preventing or reversing ID.[10] Three arms of this blinded randomized clinical trial (RCT) tested low-dose (19 mg) and medium-dose (38 mg) daily iron supplements for 8 weeks after donation against placebo pills to assess laboratory (hemoglobin, ferritin) and operational (visits, units donated, hemoglobin deferral) outcomes. Two additional arms tested an educational approach of providing donors a notification letter of low ferritin results with attendant counseling against a control group receiving only a thank you letter. In longitudinal analysis, 19 and 38 mg iron pills provided strong protection against AIS (both with odds ratios [OR] <0.2, whereas the placebo pill group worsened with an OR of 1.48). The educational results were almost as strong: a marked decrease in risk for AIS (OR = 0.43 in the notification letter group) and an increase for the letter control group (OR = 1.76). More than 70% of participants receiving the letter reported acting on its recommendations to initiate iron supplementation or to wait 6 months before donating again. Notably, iron pills did not fully eliminate ID. At the final visit, more than 30% of participants assigned to iron pills had a ferritin of less than 26 ng/mL and approximately 10% had AIS.

The HEIRS study (see **Table 1**) further illustrated the importance of iron supplementation in aligning recovery kinetics of hemoglobin and ferritin with allowable 8-week intervals. Participants were randomized to iron pills or to no treatment for 24-week observation. Daily pills with 38 mg of elemental iron shortened the hemoglobin recovery time by approximately 1.5 to 4.0 months, from an average 78 to 31 days in those with initial ferritin greater than 26 ng/mL and from 158 to 32 days in those with starting ferritin of 26 ng/mL or less. Ferritin recovery took longer but showed similar patterns: from an average more than 168 days to 21 days in those with a baseline ferritin of 26 ng/mL or less and more than 168 days to 107 days for those with an initial ferritin of more than 26 ng/mL. For two-thirds of participants not on iron, recovery of hemoglobin or ferritin to predonation levels took more than 24 weeks.

Studies on Teenage Donors in the United States

Three recent publications have addressed the iron status of teenage donors, with data derived from research endeavors, operational blood center ferritin testing, and public health surveillance efforts. The REDS-III CHILL study (see **Table 1**) enrolled a cohort of 4265 donors age 16 to 49 years, showing that 40% of donations from teen donors came from donors with a ferritin of less than 26 and 17% with a ferritin of less than 12 ng/mL.[12] Longitudinal analysis indicated that younger donors had an odds for AIS at least twice those of older donors and an odds for a ferritin of less than 26 ng/mL at least 3 times greater. In 16-year-old girls, progression to hemoglobin values of less than 12.5 g/dL was twice as likely as for females 19 to 49 years old.

These findings were reinforced by data from a large blood collector's donor safety initiative. Vassallo and colleagues[18] reported on the 16-month results for operational cutoffs (ferritin of <20 ng/mL for females and <30 ng/mL for males, defined as low ferritin) as well as ferritin of less than 12 or 26 ng/mL (termed AIS and IDE, respectively). From more than 110,000 donations tested, 9% of donors 16 to 18 years old had AIS, 32% had IDE, and 27% received low ferritin deferrals of 6 (males) or 12 months (females). A ferritin of less than 12 ng/mL was associated with sex, donation frequency, and hemoglobin. As shown in **Fig. 1**, however, although low hemoglobin is a marker for higher risk for AIS, its use—such as within 0.5 or 1.0 g/dL of the eligibility cutoffs of 12.5 or 13.0 g/dL for female and male donors—would have poor sensitivity in identifying AIS, especially in young males. Additional data from another large collector shows the steep increase in the prevalence (**Fig. 2**A) and risk (**Fig. 2**B) of ID at a higher donation frequency.[19]

Finally, Patel and colleagues[13] analyzed surveillance data from a representative national sample of females in the US. The National Health and Nutrition Surveys are conducted periodically to monitor several health indices in the US population, and the careful sampling strategy is accompanied by standardized laboratory assessments (including ferritin), questionnaire administration, and in-home ascertainment of self-reported iron and other supplement use. Here, with careful control for many covariates not routinely available to blood centers (C-reactive protein, smoking, dietary iron, iron supplementation, menses, and hormonal contraception), investigators showed donation was associated with a risk for AIS and for iron deficiency anemia (IDA) double that of nondonors 16 to 19 years old.

Studies on Adult Donors Outside the United States

Studies conducted outside the United States can reflect different donation eligibility criteria relating to minimum hemoglobin, allowable donation frequency, age restrictions, and intervals between donations; hence, estimates of prevalent ID in donors might be expected to vary. Goldman and colleagues[14] found in a representative Canadian sample (excluding Quebec province) that 17% of tested donors had a ferritin of less than 12 ng/mL and 42% had a ferritin of less than 25 ng/mL. Follow-up of tested donors found that the 2-year return rates were lower in those notified of ferritin values of less than 25 ng/mL than in donors with normal results. More impactful was the sharp decrease in units collected from repeat donors who did return to donate. Male donors gave 3 fewer units in the 2 years after notification of low ferritin results compared with the 2 years before (7.5 units vs 4.5 units) and females 2 fewer units (5 units vs 3 units).

An Australian study using a nationally representative sample used the World Health Organization cutoff of a ferritin of less than 15 ng/mL to define ID. Salvin and colleagues[16] found an overall prevalence of ID of 13.6% with a 4-fold difference between

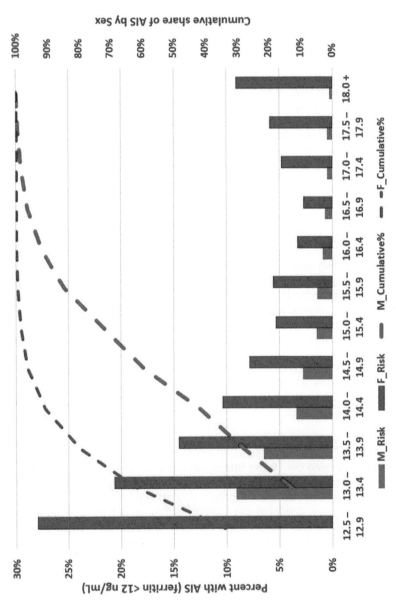

Fig. 1. Risk for and cumulative prevalence of AIS by hemoglobin interval in donors 16 to 18 years old. Hemoglobin near eligibility minimum levels (12.5 g/dL for females [F], 13.0 g/dL for males [M]) indicates higher risk for AIS. The right y-axis reflects the cumulative percentage of donations with AIS in each sex. The left y-axis reflects the cumulative percentage of donations with AIS in each sex, showing that especially for male donors a borderline hemoglobin value shows poor sensitivity for detecting AIS. (*Data from* Vassallo RR, Bravo MD, Kamel H. Ferritin testing to characterize and address iron deficiency in young donors. Transfusion 2018;58(12):2861–2867.)

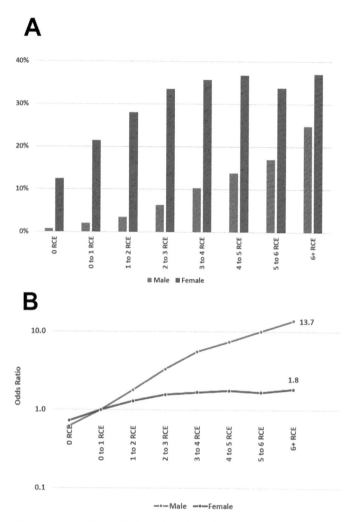

Fig. 2. Prevalence and modeled risk for AIS by donation frequency in donors 16 to 18 years old. (*A*) The prevalence of AIS is much higher in females (*red*) than males (*blue*) at any donation frequency, but the (*B*) modeled risk shows a steeper increase for males given the low baseline risk at 0 donations. RCE = red cell equivalent units donated in 2 years: whole blood = 1, double red cell donation = 2, plateletpheresis donation = 0.2 RCE.

males and females (5.4% vs 22.6%). Anemia was found in 4.2% of donors (2.3% in males vs 6.2% in females). Donation frequency was an important risk factor for ID in females but was associated with "no evident change" in males.

In the Netherlands, Baart and colleagues[17] studied 5280 accepted whole blood donors to assess for subclinical iron deficiency based on several analytes. These included serum ferritin, soluble transferrin receptor, zinc protoporphyrin, and other measures. The authors found that the prevalence might vary 4- to 5-fold depending on the laboratory assay chosen, and that the specific test yielding the low and high estimates varied by sex. Clearly, standardization of assays and caution with definitions are required when comparing one country's donor population to that of another, or to surveillance over time for a single donor population.

EVIDENCE FOR ADVERSE OUTCOMES FROM DONATION-ASSOCIATED IRON DEPLETION

Although the important causal role of blood donation for ID in blood donors is incontestable, poor documentation exists for serious adverse clinical outcomes in donors resulting from ID. The list of adverse health consequences potentially associated with ID is lengthy: fatigue, decreased exercise tolerance, cognitive dysfunction, pregnancy-related complications, pica, and restless leg syndrome. In general, the associations are stronger and more consistent for these outcomes when there is concomitant anemia; pica alone seems to have strong evidence for an association with ID in the absence of anemia.

As shown in **Box 1**, evidence for the most concerning outcomes associated with donation-related ID seems to be lacking. In large studies from Canada and Scandinavia,[20,21] where integrated national health systems allow for connection of donation behavior to health and other outcomes, the incidence of low birth weight in blood donors was not shown to be higher than in nondonors. The Danish study does indicate about a 10-g decrement in birth weight for each donation in the 3 years before pregnancy, but they are unable to ascribe higher risk for low birth weight or other outcomes from that relatively small difference.

Adverse impacts on cognitive function in blood donors has not been shown, although very few studies have addressed the subject. The INTERVAL study, a large RCT in England designed to assess the safety of donation frequencies less stringent than the statutory guidelines, assessed a large array of quality of life and donation-related symptoms, as well as cognitive function at beginning and end of 2-year follow-up. In both male and female donors, participants randomized to shorter donation intervals had lower hemoglobin and ferritin levels than those assigned to longer intervals; there was also increasing prevalence of anemia and a ferritin of less than 15 ng/mL as donation intervals were shortened (12, 14, or 16 weeks in females, 8, 10, or 12 weeks in males). Despite the hematological and iron status differences, none of 5 cognitive function assessments was associated with treatment group.

An indirect assessment of neurocognitive function was performed in Scandinavia by evaluating scholastic attainment in the children of blood donors compared with children of nondonors.[23] A "healthy donor effect" was evident in the analysis, with children

---

Box 1
Iron depletion in blood donors: assessment of potentially severe adverse outcomes

Pregnancy

- Germain and colleagues[20] found no association between donation frequency before pregnancy and low-birth weight, preterm delivery, or stillbirth
- Rigas and colleagues[21] showed lower birth weight with donation before pregnancy but of small magnitude and no higher risk for low-birth weight

Neurocognitive function

- The INTERVAL study[22] shows no difference in multiple cognitive tests at study end despite differences across treatment arms in hemoglobin and ferritin values and percentage with ID or anemia
- Rigas and colleagues[23] showed that donation frequency before pregnancy is not associated with scholastic achievement of children born to female donors.

of female donors having higher academic outcomes than those of nondonors, whereas adjusted comparisons restricted to blood donors likewise showed no association between donation frequency and academic achievement.

Any impact of donation-induced ID on the cognitive function of blood donors, whether of teenage or adult years, might be difficult to ascertain. The effects could be very subtle or of short duration. To the extent they reach the consciousness of the donor himself or herself, the concern may be self-limiting if the donor then chooses to discontinue donation. Further scientific inquiry into this topic is justified and an identified priority of the US National Institutes of Health National Heart, Lung and Blood Institute.

As noted, pica—the craving and consumption of nonfood items—is strongly associated with ID, including in blood donor studies.[24,25] Restless leg syndrome, a neurologic sensorimotor disorder characterized by uncomfortable sensations and an urge to move one's legs, is prevalent in blood donors but thus far is not shown to be associated with blood donor iron status.[24–26] Whereas the INTERVAL study reported differences in donation-related symptoms such as tiredness or breathlessness by treatment assignment, the Danish cohort did not document differences in mental or physical quality of life assessments by donor iron status.[22,27]

EVIDENCE FOR IMPACT OF IRON DEFICIENCY ON NEUROCOGNITIVE FUNCTION IN NONDONORS

Evaluating the impact of poor iron status as a single factor on neurologic, behavioral, or physiologic outcomes is a challenging endeavor. Where the treatment is oral or parenteral iron, the effect will often be to increase both hemoglobin levels and ferritin values. Even when participants fall within a population's reference range for hemoglobin, one might expect a hematopoietic response to iron if they are below their individual equilibrium value. Evidence for this relative anemia was seen in HEIRS, where 1 group of participants receiving iron returned to hemoglobin levels on average 106% of their predonation value.[11] Although a comprehensive review of the literature is beyond the scope of this article, it is worth noting that the relationship between insufficient iron and cognitive, behavioral, emotional, and other developmental outcomes has been extensively probed in infants and young children. The negative outcomes associated with iron deficiency early in life are well-established, and evidence indicates that the impact of iron deficit insults early in life may be of considerable duration, even if corrected.[28]

The impact of iron insults with onset in the adolescent or adult years has been subject to less attention, and existing studies are mostly in females of childbearing age. One of the earliest studies is a double-blinded RCT conducted by Bruner and colleagues[29] on adolescent girls in Baltimore, Maryland. The authors tested attention, memory, and learning in 78 girls with normal hemoglobin and a ferritin of less than 12 ng/mL over 8 weeks of twice daily oral iron versus placebo. At study end, none of 3 tests of attention showed significant differences by treatment, but 1 of 3 separately scored components of the Hopkins Verbal Learning Test for memory showed a difference that achieved statistical significance ($P < .02$). The variability in posttreatment scores attributed to iron was 7%, with 93% allocated to baseline performance. These findings occurred in the context of improvements in both hemoglobin (13.5 g/dL mean hemoglobin vs 12.7 g/dL mean hemoglobin) and ferritin (27 ng/mL mean ferritin vs 12 ng/mL mean ferritin) in the treatment group relative to the controls, so changes relating to ferritin improvements alone are not identifiable.

Another blinded RCT in women 18 to 35 years old randomized participants to 16-week treatment with oral iron supplements or placebo within 3 strata representing iron-sufficient controls, ID, and IDA groups.[30] The study encompassed 8 specific tasks of attention, memory, and learning, many with separate scores for performance, time to completion, and a composite score. Designed as an RCT, the study was reported as an interventional trial according to whether participants demonstrated improvement or not in hemoglobin and ferritin. At baseline, the IDA participants performed worse than both the ID and the controls on both performance and time, with the ID and controls indistinguishable. The improvements reported in longitudinal analysis on performance (for ferritin responders only) or time (for hemoglobin responders only) do not disaggregate the ID from IDA participants. A dose–response relationship was not observed for the magnitude of the cognitive change in relation to the size of hemoglobin or ferritin change.

Additional studies seeking to isolate the impact of iron deficiency without anemia on young women's cognitive function report intriguing results often focusing on executive function, described by Scott and Murray-Kolb[31] as an umbrella term capturing an array of "complex goal-directed mental operations such as planning, working memory, self-monitoring and regulation, inhibition, and volition." In a study assessing 6 measures of iron and hematological status together with 5 executive function tasks, most of the associations between iron status and executive function outcomes were null, some showed the hypothesized relationship of better performance with stronger iron status, and 1 measure indicated an unexpected negative association of worse performance with better iron status.[31] Another study looked at the relationship between 4 measures of iron status and executive function in 42 nonanemic college women.[32] The authors found no relationship between any of the measures of iron and 4 of 6 tasks representing cognitive function, and for 1 measure they found higher serum iron associated with worse performance. For 1 of 6 tasks, none of the 4 iron assays was associated with task completion or with total time on task; 1 measure (body iron) was positively associated with planning time.

In sum, the data appear interesting and may capture subtle differences, but there does not appear to be a strong and consistent signal from much of the published literature on iron deficiency without anemia.

REGULATORY STATUS AND POTENTIAL OPTIONS TO MITIGATE IRON DEPLETION
Role of the Food and Drug Administration and American Association of Blood Banks

In efforts extending more than a decade, the FDA, the federal agency providing regulatory oversight of US blood collectors, has solicited industry input on appropriate eligibility requirements for blood donors. In 2007, the FDA published proposed rules in the Federal Register and sought comment on considerations of safety and blood availability related to lowering the minimum hemoglobin for female donors (from 12.5 g/dL to 12.0 g/dL), continuing to collect from male donors at the below normal cutoff of 12.5 g/dL, and to adopting a "more stringent inter-donation interval."[33] Subsequent meetings of the agency's Blood Products Advisory Committee in 2008 and 2010 heard discussions about hemoglobin distributions in healthy individuals, appropriate hemoglobin measurement, the prevalence of low ferritin in United States and other countries' donors, and considerations of supply under modified eligibility criteria.[34,35] The committee unanimously agreed in 2008 that ID in blood donors was cause for concern, but at both meetings definitive action on donation intervals was not recommended pending final results from RISE (see **Table 1**) and data presented indicating a potentially sizable impact on availability if 12- or 16-week intervals were adopted. The final rule published in May 2015[36] increased the minimum hemoglobin for male donors to 13.0 g/dL and contemplated allowing the collection of blood from female donors with a hemoglobin as low as 12.0 g/dL as long as additional steps to ensure donor safety were undertaken and were approved by FDA.

A third Blood Products Advisory Committee meeting in November 2016 added momentum to accumulating concerns on ID with presentation of data on high-school age donors.[37] CHILL data showed that more than 40% of donations from donors 16 to 18 years old in the REDS-III study had a ferritin of less than 26 ng/mL and that the ferritin distributions in first-time donors were different between younger donors and adult controls 19 to 49 years old. The committee unanimously acknowledged the susceptibility of teen donors to ID and recommended further study as well as transparency in communications with teen donors and their parents.

The accreditor of US blood collectors, AABB (formerly the American Association of Blood Banks), has played an active role in communicating updates and recommendations to its membership. After the publication of the initial RISE results,[7] the AABB released an Association Bulletin in 2012 characterizing subpopulations of donors considered at risk for ID with recommendations for preventing or reversing ID in donors.[38] These options are summarized in **Box 2** and detailed here, but none was mandatory or integrated into a new standard required for blood bank accreditation. After the presentation of CHILL data at Blood Products Advisory Committee, an updated bulletin to membership was released in March 2017.[39] AABB Association Bulletin #17-02 took a stronger tone and, notably, explicitly recommended limiting high school age donors to a single donation per year unless other safety measures were undertaken. This recommendation was not binding, but it reflected a clear posture that sufficient evidence had accumulated that blood centers should proceed with 1 or more mitigation approaches in at least their youngest donors.

In May 2017, AABB convened an expert panel to apply a risk-based decision-making framework to assessing the problem of ID in blood donors. This group was tasked with characterizing the problem of ID in donors, assessing the evidence for safety, and

---

Box 2
Mitigation of ID

Donation restrictions

- Pros: limited complexity and implementation cost (eg, to restrict by age or to lengthen donation intervals)

- Cons: unknown but potentially sizable impact on blood collections; may not target group(s) of high concern

Ferritin testing

- Pros: direct assessment of iron status; may stimulate donor response more effectively than generalized messaging

- Cons: cost of both the assay and donor replacement; no consensus on optimal cutoff for donor eligibility or donor management considerations

Iron supplementation

- Pros: aligns recovery times of hemoglobin and ferritin with allowable donation intervals for most donors

- Cons: cost; logistics; contraindications for some donors; uncertain compliance; legal implications

evaluating alternative approaches with attendant implications. This process engaged heavily with stakeholders on the "source" end (parents, high school staff, young donors), the eventual users (clinicians, transfusion services, patient advocacy groups), and public health specialists at local and national levels. The report, which has been accepted by the AABB Board of Directors, acknowledges that the evidence for harm from ID in young donors is lacking, but on a precautionary basis urges blood center action to mitigate against the potential for impact on cognitive function.[40] At the moment, no consensus optimal approach exists. Most likely no single approach will be uniformly embraced, given the widely disparate financial and logistic considerations based on geography and size of US blood collectors. Two large collectors accounting for approximately one-half of US collections implemented ferritin testing for its 16- to 18-year-old donors, but some controversy exists about whether the theoretic harm justifies potentially costly mitigation strategies that also make it more challenging to collect the blood to meet patient needs.[41]

Mitigation Option 1: Restrict Donation Frequency or Eligibility

In principle, restricting donation frequency might be attractive given the potential for relatively simple configuration changes to the blood center computer system. These could range from merely increasing the minimum age to 17 or 18 years old to redefining the minimum interval between single-unit red cell donations from 8 to 12 or 16 weeks.

There are 2 primary drawbacks to restricting donation frequency or eligibility. First, the impact on collections could be meaningful, in the mid to high single digits depending on configuration. One recent report indicates that 16- to 18-year-olds account for as much as 14% of collections with much of the increase in recent years driven by more donations from 16 year olds.[2] Removing them from eligibility, or restricting them to one donation per year as recommended by AABB Association Bulletin #17-02 could have cascading effects requiring significant restructuring of a blood center's recruitment plans. Excess capacity in collections has been nearly eliminated, with a narrow margin between units collected and units transfused being seen on an annual basis.[1]

The second major concern is that mitigation of ID is likely to be modest unless intervals are extended to an extent that blood component availability is seriously compromised. A simulation study showed that intervals of 12 or 16 weeks would still leave uncorrected approximately 80% of the existing iron deficiency in blood donor populations.[9] The reason for this is evident from the HEIRS study, which showed that for both hemoglobin and ferritin, two-thirds of donors did not return to a predonation baseline within 24 weeks if they were not supplementing with iron.[11] Similar findings have been reported from Europe.[42,43]

Mitigation Option 2: Add a Direct Measure of Iron Status

Direct assessment of donor iron is increasingly considered worthy of pursuit, with 2 national blood collectors having begun testing its teenage donors.[18,19] Although many assays have been evaluated,[17] the current evidence suggests that serum or plasma ferritin is the single best test to determine the iron levels of a blood donor. A current limitation in the United States is the lack of a licensed point-of-care assay allowing for ferritin determination at the blood drive. If such a test became available, it could potentially be integrated into donor eligibility algorithms or used for donor messaging and management, at a blood center's discretion or if eventually required by AABB or by FDA. Which donors to test, what ferritin level to use as a cutoff, and the specific action following a low result might be configured in a multitude of ways.

Ferritin testing has its own downsides, too. The cost is not limited to 1-time computer system changes, but rather is directly related to the number of donors tested. As shown by available results,[18,19] depending on where one sets the bar, the share of donors with low ferritin results may indeed be large. Replacing these donors lost to the donor pool, at least temporarily, adds to the overall cost of a ferritin program. To the extent donors self-remove permanently, the loss may be greater. Multiple studies have documented a deterrent effect of deferral (even short term), and the recent study by Goldman and colleagues[15] in Canada show an average decline in collections of 3 units in males and 2 units in females 2 years after notification of low ferritin results. In contrast, the STRIDE study showed enhanced donation productivity from donors getting a letter with their low ferritin values and recommendations to wait 6 months for their next donation or start taking iron. Whether these encouraging results from a very select, motivated donor population will apply more broadly remains an open question.

Mitigation Option 3: Iron Supplementation

The benefits of iron supplementation are obvious in the accelerated recovery kinetics for hemoglobin and ferritin shown in HEIRS.[11] The low-dose formulations currently available show good tolerability, and in STRIDE the incidence of side effects (most notably gastrointestinal symptoms) was the same in the 2 groups assigned to iron pills as to the placebo group.[10] Although blood centers recommend well-balanced diets with plenty of iron-rich foods to their donors, expert opinion and HEIRS results emphasize the insufficiency of dietary iron alone to return many donors to an iron-replete state.[11,40]

The challenges to iron supplementation include financial costs associated with purchasing, stocking, and distributing iron pills. Some donors may have contraindications for the ingestion of exogenous iron pills, whether owing to risk for hereditary hemochromatosis or other conditions. Compliance on donors' part remains untested in an operational context, outside the research setting. Finally, legal analysis conducted by the risk-based decision-making work group convened by the AABB indicated that state laws on the practice of medicine might cover the distribution of iron pills.[40] The implications of a "practice of medicine" determination would, for many blood centers, be sufficiently onerous to eliminate consideration of distributing iron in a blood center setting.

Alternative strategies could be enhanced education regarding the need for iron to maintain fitness for regular donation. Evidence is limited outside the research context, but it seems that only 21% of donors report taking iron either as a multivitamin or a separate iron pill.[44] Blood centers could partner with pharmacies to distribute coupons for discounted or free iron pills, but this has not been tested and may have legal implications, too.

SUMMARY

A large proportion of blood donors in the United States and other countries develop ID. This is particularly true for frequent donors, premenopausal females, and donors 16 to 18 years old. The clinical outcomes resulting from ID in nonanemic blood donors remain for the most part poorly documented. The most worrisome outcomes relating to cognitive function or to fetal outcomes have not been shown in blood donor studies to date. In nondonor populations, the available evidence on cognitive outcomes and ID without anemia is suggestive but not conclusive. These data are of considerable interest and bear monitoring as research progresses. Meanwhile, blood centers should communicate clearly with their donors and through this relationship strive to limit the development and progression of iron deficiency.

ACKNOWLEDGMENTS

The author has received support from the National Heart Lung and Blood Institute for the REDS-II and REDS-III contracts (numbered HHSN268200447169C and HHSN268201100006I, respectively) and grant award 1R01HL105809, which supported the STRIDE study.

REFERENCES

1. Ellingson KD, Sapiano MRP, Haass KA, et al. Continued decline in blood collection and transfusion in the United States - 2015. Transfusion 2017;57(Suppl 2):1588–98.
2. Eder AF, Crowder LA, Steele WR. Teenage blood donation: demographic trends, adverse reactions, and iron balance. ISBT Sci Ser 2017;12:395–400.
3. Finch CA, Cook JD, Labbe RF, et al. Effect of blood donation on iron stores as evaluated by serum ferritin. Blood 1977;50:441–7.
4. Simon TL, Garry PJ, Hooper EM. Iron stores in blood donors. J Am Med Assoc 1981;245:2038–43.
5. Milman N, Sondergaard M. Iron stores in male blood donors evaluated by serum ferritin. Transfusion 1984;24:464–8.
6. Bianco C, Brittenham G, Gilcher RO, et al. Maintaining iron balance in women blood donors of childbearing age: summary of a workshop. Transfusion 2002; 42(6):798–805.
7. Cable RG, Glynn SA, Kiss JE, et al, NHLBI Retrovirus Epidemiology Donor Study-II. Iron deficiency in blood donors: analysis of enrollment data from the REDS-II Donor Iron Status Evaluation (RISE) study. Transfusion 2011;51:511–22.
8. Cable RG, Glynn SA, Kiss JE, et al. Iron deficiency in blood donors: the REDS-II Donor Iron Status Evaluation (RISE) study. Transfusion 2012;52:702–11.
9. Spencer BR, Johnson B, Wright DJ, et al. Potential impact on blood availability and donor iron status of changes to donor hemoglobin cutoff and interdonation intervals. Transfusion 2016;56(8):1994–2004.
10. Mast AE, Bialkowski W, Bryant BJ, et al. A randomized, blinded, placebo-controlled trial of education and iron supplementation for mitigation of iron deficiency in regular blood donors. Transfusion 2016;56:1588–97.
11. Kiss JE, Brambilla D, Glynn SA, et al. Oral iron supplementation after blood donation: a randomized clinical trial. JAMA 2015;6:575–83.
12. Spencer BR, Bialkowski W, Creel DV, et al. Elevated risk for iron depletion in high-school age donors. Transfusion 2019. https://doi.org/10.1111/trf.15133.
13. Patel EU, White JL, Bloch EM, et al. Association of blood donation with iron deficiency among adolescent and adult females in the United States: a nationally representative study. Transfusion 2019. https://doi.org/10.1111/trf.15179.
14. Goldman M, Uzicanin S, Osmond L, et al. A large national study of ferritin testing in Canadian blood donors. Transfusion 2017;57:564–70.
15. Goldman M, Uzicanin S, Osmond L, et al. Two-year follow-up of donors in a large national study of ferritin testing. Transfusion 2018;58:2868–73.
16. Salvin HE, Pasricha SR, Marks DC, et al. Iron deficiency in blood donors: a national cross-sectional study. Transfusion 2014;54:2434–44.
17. Baart AM, van Noord A, Vergouwe Y, et al. High prevalence of subclinical iron deficiency in whole blood donors not deferred for low hemoglobin. Transfusion 2013;53:1670–7.
18. Vassallo RR, Bravo MD, Kamel H. Ferritin testing to characterize and address iron deficiency in young donors. Transfusion 2018;58:2861–7.

19. Spencer BR, Haynes JM, Rambaud ML. Ferritin testing to mitigate risk for iron depletion in high school blood donors. Transfusion 2018;58(Suppl 2):49A.

20. Germain M, Delage G, Robillard P, et al. The association between frequency of blood donation and the occurrence of low birthweight, preterm delivery, and still-birth: a retrospective cohort study. Transfusion 2016;56:2760–7.

21. Rigas AS, Pedersen OB, Sorensen E, et al. Frequent blood donation and offspring birth weight—a next-generation association? Transfusion 2019;59:995–1001.

22. Di Angelantonio E, Thompson SG, Kaptoge S, et al. Efficiency and safety of vary-ing the frequency of whole blood donation (INTERVAL): a randomised trial of 45000 donors. Lancet 2017;390(10110):2360–71.

23. Rigas AS, Pedersen OB, Rostgaard K, et al. Frequent blood donation and offspring scholastic attainment: an assessment of long-term consequences of prenatal iron deficiency. Transfusion 2019. https://doi.org/10.1111/trf.15193.

24. Bryant BJ, Yau YY, Arceo SM, et al. Ascertainment of iron deficiency and deple-tion in blood donors through screening questions for pica and restless legs syn-drome. Transfusion 2013;53:1637–44.

25. Spencer B, Kleinman S, Wright D, et al. Restless legs syndrome, pica and iron status in blood donors. Transfusion 2013;53:1645–52.

26. Didriksen M, Rigas AS, Allen RP, et al. Prevalence of restless legs syndrome and associated factors in an otherwise healthy population: results from the Danish Blood Donor Study. Sleep Med 2017;36:55–61.

27. Rigas AS, Pedersen OB, Sorensen CJ, et al. No association between iron status and self-reported health-related quality of life in 16,375 Danish blood donors: re-sults from the Danish Blood Donor Study. Transfusion 2015;55:1752–6.

28. Georgieff MK. Iron assessment to protect the developing brain. Am J Clin Nutr 2017;106(Suppl):1588S–93S.

29. Bruner AB, Joffe A, Duggan AK, et al. Randomised study of cognitive effects of iron supplementation in non-anaemic iron-deficient adolescent girls. Lancet 1996;348:992–6.

30. Murray-Kolb LE, Beard JL. Iron treatment normalizes cognitive functioning in young women. Am J Clin Nutr 2007;85:778–876.

31. Scott SP, Murray-Kolb LE. Iron status is associated with performance on execu-tive functioning tasks in nonanemic young women. J Nutr 2016;146:30–7.

32. Blanton CA, Green MW, Kretsch MJ. Body iron is associated with cognitive exec-utive planning function in college women. Br J Nutr 2013;109:906–13.

33. Food and Drug Administration. Requirements for human blood and blood components intended for transfusion or for further manufacturing use, 21 CFR Sect. 606, 610, 630, 640, 660, 820, 1270 (2007). Proposed rule. Available at: https://www.govinfo.gov/content/pkg/FR-2007-11-08/pdf/E7-21565.pdf. Accessed April 8, 2019.

34. Food and Drug Administration, Center for Biologics Evaluation and Research. Blood Products Advisory Committee, 92nd Meeting, September 10, 2008, meeting minutes. Available at: https://wayback.archive-it.org/7993/201704040 42923/https://www.fda.gov/ohrms/dockets/ac/08/minutes/2008-4379M.html. Ac-cessed April 8, 2019.

35. Food and Drug Administration Center for Biologics Evaluation and Research. Blood Products Advisory Committee. July 27, 2010, transcript. Available at: https://wayback.archive-it.org/7993/20170113201602/http://www.fda.gov/down loads/AdvisoryCommittees/CommitteesMeetingMaterials/BloodVaccinesand OtherBiologics/BloodProductsAdvisoryCommittee/UCM225389.pdf. Accessed April 8, 2019.

36. Food and Drug Administration. Requirements for human blood and blood compo-nents intended for transfusion or for further manufacturing use, 21 CFR Sect. 606, 610, 630, 640, 660, 820, 1270 (2007). Final rule. Available at: https://www.govinfo.gov/content/pkg/FR-2015-05-22/pdf/2015-12228.pdf. Accessed April 8, 2019.

37. Food and Drug Administration, Center for Biologics Evaluation and Research. Blood Products Advisory Committee, 92nd Meeting, November 17. 2016, meeting minutes. Available at: https://www.fda.gov/downloads/AdvisoryCommittees/CommitteesMeetingMaterials/BloodVaccinesandOtherBiologics/BloodProductsAdvisoryCommittee/UCM582198.pdf. Accessed April 8, 2019.

38. AABB. Association bulletin #12-03: strategies to monitor, limit or prevent iron deficiency in blood donors. Available at: http://www.aabb.org/programs/publications/bulletins/Pages/abobsolete.aspx. Accessed April 12, 2019.

39. AABB. Association bulletin #17-02: updated strategies to limit or prevent iron deficiency in blood donors. Available at: http://www.aabb.org/programs/publications/bulletins/Pages/ab18-01.aspx. Accessed April 12, 2019.

40. AABB. AABB donor iron deficiency risk-based decision-making assessment report: report of the ad hoc iron deficiency working group. 2019. Available at: http://www.aabb.org/tm/Documents/AABB-Donor-Iron-Deficiency-RBDM-Assessment-Report.pdf. Accessed April 8, 2019.

41. Vassallo RR. Donor iron depletion: beneficial or burdensome? Transfusion 2019. https://doi.org/10.1111/trf.15282.

42. Schotten N, Pasker-de Jong PC, Moretti D, et al. The donation interval of 56 days requires extension to 180 days for whole blood donors to recover from changes in iron metabolism. Blood 2016;128:2185–8.

43. Baart AM, van den Hurk K, de Kort WL. Minimum donation intervals should be reconsidered to decrease low hemoglobin deferral in whole blood donors: an observational study. Transfusion 2015;55:2641–4.

44. Cable RG, Spencer BR. Iron supplementation by blood donors: demographics, patterns of use, and motivation. Transfusion 2019. [Epub ahead of print].

Impact of Novel Monoclonal Antibody Therapeutics on Blood Bank Pretransfusion Testing

Zhen Mei, MD[a], Geoffrey D. Wool, MD, PhD[b],*

KEYWORDS

- Immunohematology • Monoclonal antibody therapy • CD47 • CD38
- Pretransfusion testing

KEY POINTS

- The role of monoclonal antibodies is expanding in oncology and some monoclonal antibody agents may interfere with pretransfusion testing owing to reagent red blood cell expression of target antigens.
- Anti-CD38 agents do not interfere with blood group typing, but cause pan-reactivity during indirect antiglobulin testing, which may mask a potentially clinically significant antibody.
- Wide variability is demonstrated with different anti-CD47/SIRPα agents, with some agents more significantly interfering with compatibility testing; future studies are needed to further characterize these agents.
- Accurate medication lists, including trial therapeutics, must be promptly communicated to the blood bank to facilitate rational sample workup and timely delivery of safe blood products.

CASE

A woman with a history of B-cell lymphoma (not otherwise specified), status post stem cell transplant, presents with anemia. Pretransfusion testing at the hospital reports an unresolvable pan-agglutinin using automated gel methodology. Therefore, the patient sample is referred to an immunohematology reference laboratory for additional workup. Her transfusion history includes receipt of 2 units of packed red blood cells (RBCs) in the previous month after a negative antibody screen. No medication history is provided.

Disclosure Statement: The authors have nothing to disclose; they declare there are no conflicts of interest or disclosures relevant to the article submitted to *Hematology/Oncology Clinics of North America*.
[a] University of Chicago Medicine, 5841 South Maryland Avenue, AMB S339, MC 3083, Chicago, IL 60637, USA; [b] Department of Pathology, University of Chicago, 5841 South Maryland Avenue, AMB S339, MC 3083, Chicago, IL 60637, USA
* Corresponding author.
E-mail address: geoffrey.wool@uchospitals.edu

Immunohematology reference laboratory workup revealed the following:

1. ABO typing showed a discrepancy with additional plasma reactivity: forward-typed as group B+ and back-typed as group O.
2. Antibody panels performed with tube technique using polyethylene glycol and low ionic strength saline demonstrated strong pan-reactivity with a negative autocontrol. Further panels also demonstrated strong pan-reactivity, including ficin treated cells and phenotypically matched cells treated with dithiothreitol (DTT) or glycine acid EDTA.
3. A polyspecific direct antiglobulin test performed in tube was negative. An eluate demonstrated strong positivity with all the cells tested with the last wash confirmed to be negative.
4. Serial titrations of the patient plasma tested against a phenotype matched cell demonstrated reactivity at antihuman globulin (AHG) phase even at 1:4096.
5. Plasma showed continued strong reactivity with rare red cells lacking high-frequency antigens, including Lan, Vel, PP1Pk (Tja), En[a], I, H, Cs[a], and Co[a].
6. Allo-adsorption with ficin-treated human RBC stroma resolved the forward and back type discrepancy (confirmed as B+), but still could not resolve the plasma reactivity.

The resolution of this interference required additional information from the ordering hospital: a medication history was provided and it was discovered that this patient had been receiving an anti-CD47 agent. This extended, unfruitful workup is representative of the difficulties that can be encountered during pretransfusion testing in the setting of immunotherapeutics that interfere with pretransfusion testing.

INTRODUCTION

The modern era of monoclonal antibody (mAb) therapeutic agents became a possibility when Köhler and Milstein[1] first described a process to manufacture antibodies of predetermined specificity in 1975. The concluding thought, "Such [hybridoma] cultures could be valuable for medical and industrial use," merely scratched the surface of the potential of this technology, for which the 2 were awarded the Nobel Prize in 1984.[2] The first mAb to be approved by the US Food and Drug Administration (FDA) for clinical use was muromonab (OKT3, anti-CD3) for the prevention of graft rejection in kidney transplant recipients in 1985.[3] In 1997, rituximab (anti-CD20) became the first mAb to gain FDA approval for the treatment of an oncologic disease.[3,4]

The pharmacologic specificity of mAbs has spurred great interest in drug development; in 2000, a mere quarter century after the manufacturing of mAbs was first described, a survey suggested that more than one-quarter of all therapeutics in development were mAbs.[3] A review in 2018 listed 23 mAbs approved for the treatment of various solid and hematologic malignancies.[5]

The mAbs can variably interfere with clinical laboratory testing. Serum protein electrophoresis and immunofixation show mAb interference regardless of the specificity of the mAb, by the detection of a paraprotein that could falsely label the patient as having a monoclonal gammopathy.[6,7]

Outside of serum protein electrophoresis and immunofixation, interference with clinical laboratory testing by mAbs depends on the specificity of the mAb. Flow cytometric detection of malignant cell populations can be hindered by mAb interference.[8] Any mAbs that bind to antigens present on reagent RBCs and/or patient RBCs will cause interference with pretransfusion testing. That interference is the subject of this review.

Pretransfusion testing involves 2 stages:

1. ABO/RhD typing performed at immediate spin/room temperature
2. Screening for unexpected antibodies at 37°C and at the AHG stage (the indirect antiglobulin test [IAT])

Blood banks and immunohematology reference laboratory services started to notice mAbs when patient samples began showing significant interference, typically behaving similarly to a warm autoantibody or an alloantibody to a high incidence antigen. Two classes of mAbs, anti-CD38 and anti-CD47 agents, have demonstrated significant interference with pretransfusion testing (**Fig. 1**). This is due to the presence of CD38 and CD47 epitopes on the RBC surface.

One anti-CD38 mAb (daratumumab, Janssen Biotech, PA) is FDA approved for use in myeloma. Other anti-CD38 and anti-CD47 mAbs are in trial for use in hematolymphoid malignancies and solid tumors. Daratumumab has also been used off-label for autoimmune disorders.

The use of these mAb agents in the setting of hematolymphoid malignancy ensures a patient population with a frequent baseline hypoproliferative anemia. Additionally, because anti-CD38 and anti-CD47 mAbs both recognize epitopes that are present on RBCs, they both have the potential to cause a degree of immune hemolytic anemia. Baseline anemia, possible drug-related anemia exacerbation, and significant delays for compatibility testing is an unhappy trifecta.

Here, the authors provide a discussion of the physiology of CD38 and CD47, a list of available mAbs directed against those epitopes, the currently published pharmacologic properties of anti-CD38 and anti-CD47 mAbs, and a description of their interference pattern and the methods described to resolve their interference. The description of interference patterns is well-described for daratumumab. For the other anti-CD38 and anti-CD47 agents currently in trial, the published literature is much less robust. We describe that literature, as well as our personal experiences.

ANTI-CD38 AGENTS
CD38 Physiology

CD38, or cyclic ADP ribose hydrolase, is a widely expressed transmembrane glycoprotein found on hematolymphoid cell membranes.[9] CD38 has multiple cellular functions, including cell signaling and adhesion.[10]

Although it is expressed on many hematolymphoid cells,[9] CD38 is very highly expressed on plasma cells, allowing it to be a target of mAb therapy in myeloma. Anti-CD38 agents seem to inhibit malignant plasma cell proliferation by both activating intracellular apoptosis machinery and extracellular immune-mediated cell lysis and phagocytosis.[11] Of relevance to this discussion, the surface of erythrocytes contains a relatively small number of CD38 molecules.[12,13]

Available Anti-CD38 Agents

There is 1 FDA approved anti-CD38 mAb in clinical use (daratumumab), which is approved for the treatment of plasma cell myeloma. Daratumumab, a human IgG1 kappa mAb, was first approved in 2015 for relapsed and refractory plasma cell myeloma; the approval was broadened in 2018 to include initial treatment of transplant-ineligible myeloma. Additional anti-CD38 agents[14] are in clinical trials (**Table 1** and clinicaltrials.gov).

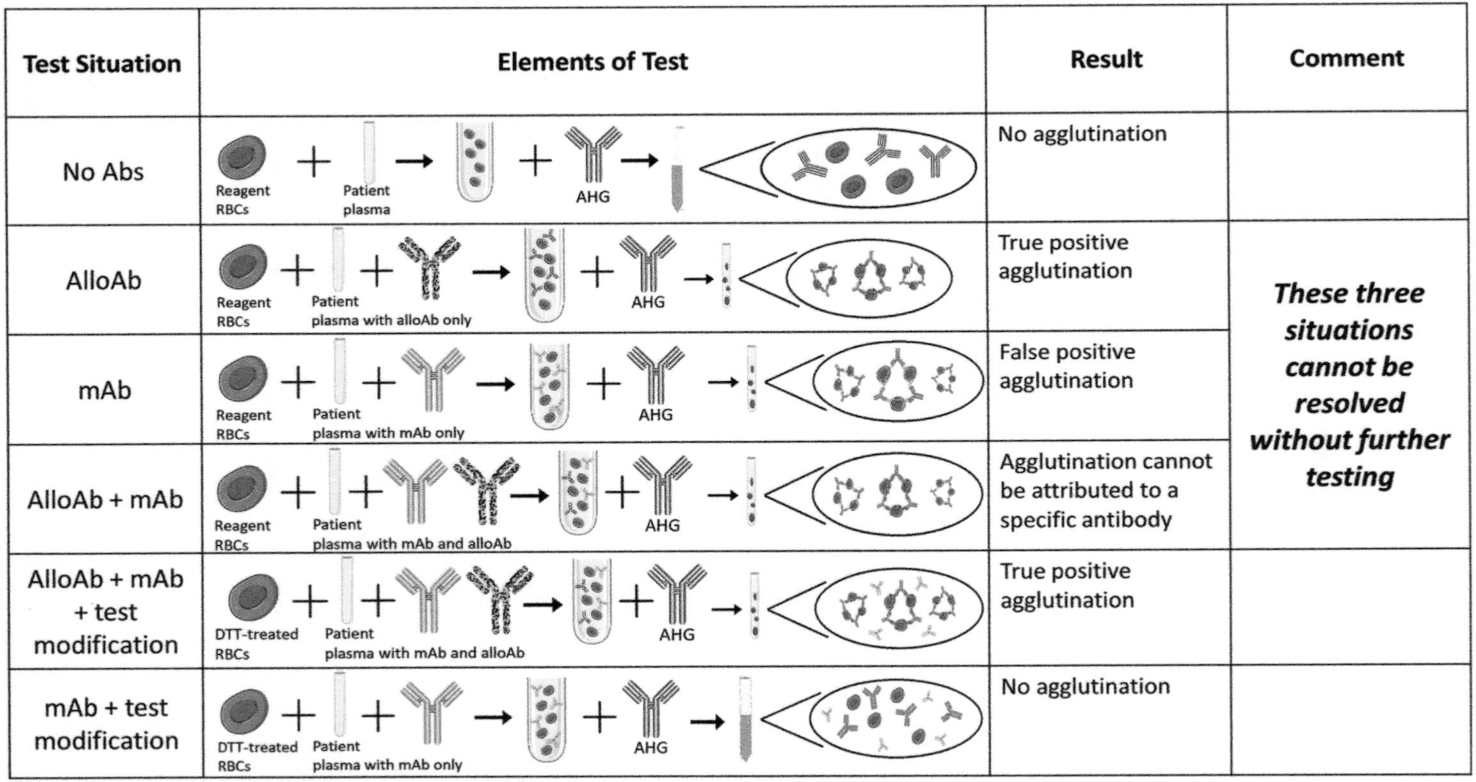

Test Situation	Elements of Test	Result	Comment
No Abs	Reagent RBCs + Patient plasma + AHG	No agglutination	
AlloAb	Reagent RBCs + Patient plasma with alloAb only + AHG	True positive agglutination	*These three situations cannot be resolved without further testing*
mAb	Reagent RBCs + Patient plasma with mAb only + AHG	False positive agglutination	
AlloAb + mAb	Reagent RBCs + Patient plasma with mAb and alloAb + AHG	Agglutination cannot be attributed to a specific antibody	
AlloAb + mAb + test modification	DTT-treated RBCs + Patient plasma with mAb and alloAb + AHG	True positive agglutination	
mAb + test modification	DTT-treated RBCs + Patient plasma with mAb only + AHG	No agglutination	

Fig. 1. Pretransfusion compatibility testing patterns. Pretransfusion testing is generally performed with red cell agglutination as the end point. This image shows the IAT, which is used for detection of unexpected anti-RBC antibodies. When no agglutination occurs, there is no antibody present; conversely, when agglutination occurs, further investigation into the possibility of and the specificity of an alloantibody progresses. When therapeutic mAbs are present, they hide the effect of any possible true alloantibody presence in the patient's serum. The mAb represented here is anti-CD38. (*Modified from* Chari A, Arinsburg S, Jagannath S, et al. Blood transfusion management and transfusion-related outcomes in daratumumab-treated patients with relapsed or refractory multiple myeloma. Clin Lymphoma Myeloma Leuk 2018;18(1):45; with permission.)

Table 1			
Anti-CD38 agents currently in clinical trials			
Company and Name of Agent	Trial Identifier(s)	Agent Properties	Trial Indication(s)
Sanofi Isatuximab (SAR650984)	NCT02990338 NCT03275285 NCT03319667 NCT03499808 NCT03617731	Human anti-CD38 IgG1 antibody	Plasma cell myeloma; relapsed/refractory primary amyloidosis
MorphoSys AG MOR03087 (MOR202)	NCT01421186	Human anti-CD38 antibody	Relapsed/refractory plasma cell myeloma
Glenmark Pharmaceuticals S.A. GBR 1342	NCT03309111	Monoclonal bispecific anti-CD3/anti-CD38 antibody	Plasma cell myeloma
Takeda (Millennium Pharmaceuticals, Inc.) TAK-079	NCT03439280 NCT03724916	Human anti-CD38 IgG1 antibody	Systemic lupus erythematosus; relapsed/refractory plasma cell myeloma

This list is not comprehensive, but representative of more recent and advanced clinical trials.

Pharmacology of Anti-CD38 Agents

When daratumumab binds to plasma cell surface CD38, it activates multiple immune mechanisms, including complement-dependent cytotoxicity, antibody-dependent cellular cytotoxicity, antibody-dependent phagocytosis, and induction of apoptosis.[15,16]

Phase II studies showed daratumumab monotherapy efficacy at 16 mg/kg, which correlated with 99% saturation of the CD38 target.[15,17] A circulating daratumumab concentration of 2.0 g/L has been categorized as super-pharmacologic.[18]

Anti-CD38 agents bind CD38 on the RBC surface and may therefore cause splenic clearance of antibody-coated erythrocytes and extravascular hemolysis.[13,19] The resultant decrease in hemoglobin is generally mild and not severe enough to be the sole cause of a patient's transfusion requirement.

Elimination of daratumumab is nonlinear; as the dosage and administration frequency increased, the half-life increased and the clearance rate decreased.[15,17] The average length of time that daratumumab can be detected varies: detection by pretransfusion testing continues for months after the patient has discontinued treatment.[20–22] Daratumumab can, exceptionally, remain detectable for up to 9 months,[22] but generally disappears within 5 to 6 months after treatment.[20]

Effects of Anti-CD38 Agents on Pretransfusion Testing

There is no noticeable effect of daratumumab on patient ABO/RhD typing. This is likely due the inability of IgG daratumumab molecules to cause direct agglutination without secondary potentiation by AHG.

Patients treated with daratumumab show pan-reactivity in the IAT (see **Fig. 1**), because CD38 is ubiquitously expressed on RBCs. The autocontrol and direct antiglobulin tests, however, are only variably positive.[21,23] This may be due to loss of RBC CD38 expression after daratumumab treatment, as has been described.[24,25] Eluates are also variable and can reveal either a pan-agglutinin[26] or are negative.[21]

Given a pan-agglutinin in the eluate, this result could suggest a warm autoantibody in a patient who was not recently transfused. If an eluate is not performed and the autocontrol is negative, a high-titer, low avidity–like antibody could be suspected based on the IAT.[23] In addition to the mistaken identification of these pan-agglutinins, the presence of anti-CD38 often prevents adequate rule-outs and may mask the presence of a true alloantibody. Cross-matches performed on samples with daratumumab will be positive as well, unless the donor cells are DTT treated.[14,21,27]

The effects of daratumumab on pretransfusion testing are summarized in **Table 2**. There is no current published literature or specific guidance on isatuximab and MOR202, but preliminary studies have shown that these agents exert similar interferences and, therefore, may represent a class-wide effect, rather than limited specifically to daratumumab.[19]

Table 2
Representative pretransfusion compatibility testing results for daratumumab

	Patient Results Before Anti-CD38 Therapy	Patient Results Post Anti-CD38 Therapy	Presence of Interference?
ABO/Rh typing	A+	A+	No
Antibody screen (IAT)	Negative	Pan-reactive positive	Yes
Autocontrol	Negative	Negative/positive	Possible
Direct antiglobulin test	Negative	Negative/positive	Possible
Eluate	Not performed	Negative/pan-agglutinin	Possible

Resolution of Interference

When the initial pan-agglutinin pattern was observed, many blood banks attempted to adsorb the pan-agglutinin away. However, owing to the high titers of anti-CD38 antibodies present in the patient plasma and the fairly low number of CD38 molecules on the RBC surface, adsorption was not effective when performed in the typical fashion. Other ways to resolve this interference were subsequently developed[19,22,23,27–30]:

1. DTT or 2-aminoethylisothiouronium treatment of screening panel red cells
   Pros
   - Reduces a disulfide linkage in the CD38 antigen, therefore denaturing the protein and destroying the epitope recognized by the anti-CD38 antibody
   - May be used for any anti-CD38 antibody because this affects the target antigen
   - DTT is a common reagent that is already found in many blood banks
   Cons
   - Destroys and denatures RBC antigens containing a disulfide linkage, including the clinically relevant Kell antigens, along with other minor blood groups, including Dombrock, Indian, JMH, Scianna, Knops, Cromer, Landsteiner-Weiner, Lutheran, MER2, AnWj, and Cartwright antigens
   - Time intensive to DTT treat the panel, wash, and store in stabilizing storage solution
2. Soluble CD38
   Pros
   - Binds to and neutralizes free anti-CD38 antibodies, saturating the binding sites, preventing them from binding to CD38 epitopes on RBC screening cells
   - Can be quickly added to patient sample before testing
   Cons
   - Expensive reagent; not widely available
   - Must be added in excess to ensure neutralization of any remaining anti-CD38 antibodies

3. Anti-idiotype antibody

Pros

- Binds to Fab portion of free anti-CD38 antibodies, saturating the binding sites, preventing them from binding to screening cells
- Can be quickly added to patient sample before testing

Cons

- Expensive reagent; not widely available
- A separate reagent may be required for each anti-CD38 mAb, because they may not all be recognized by the same anti-idiotype antibody

4. Use of cord blood as reagent RBCs for IAT[31]

Pros

- Low CD38 expression on the surface of these cells, preventing anti-CD38 antibodies from interfering
- Can rule out all antigens expressed in normal density on neonatal RBC; this includes Kell

Cons

- May be used for screening, but impractical to make an antibody identification panel using only cord blood cells
- Highly effort intensive to maintain an adequate supply of in-date and typed cord blood cells

Overall, the most common solution used by transfusion services for anti-CD38 interference is DTT-treated reagent red cells (typically treated with 0.1–0.2 mol/L DTT, as described in Judd and associate's Methods in Immunohematology[32]). If the results of an antibody screen with DTT cells remain positive, the patient likely has underlying allo-antibodies or auto-antibodies, in addition to daratumumab. Because DTT destroys the clinically relevant Kell antigens, it is useful to genotype or phenotype the patient before treatment; if the patient is known to be Kell antigen positive, the presence of any subsequent anti-Kell can be ruled out by phenotype/genotype. However, if typing was not performed or the patient is Kell antigen negative, the patient should be transfused with compatible Kell antigen-negative blood owing to the inability to properly rule out the presence of anti-K. This is typically accomplished with little difficulty, because K is a relatively low-frequency antigen.

At University of Chicago Medicine, the authors included non-daratumumab patient samples with alloantibodies in our validation of DTT-treated panels (**Table 3**). In this setting, the authors confirmed that almost all antibodies with specificities outside of the Kell system were detectable with DTT-treated reagent red cells, with 1 exception. They noted the inability of patient samples with newly developed anti-E (within 6 months of initial identification) to reliably react with E-positive DTT-treated reagent red cells; 3 of 15 tested samples (20%) with a known anti-E alloantibody were not detected with DTT-treated reagent red cells. Of the 3 nondetected anti-E antibodies with DTT-treated red cells, the time elapsed since antibody detection ranged from 0 to 5 months (mean, 1.7 months; median, 0 months). In contrast, the detected anti-E antibodies had a mean time from detection of 30 months (median, 4 months). (Marilyn A. Stewart, MS Ed MT(ASCP)SBB, unpublished data, 2017). This loss of detectability of nascent anti-E has not been described by others.[33] Although the mechanism for this finding is unclear, it is our policy at University of Chicago Medicine that, for those patients who have antibody rule-outs performed with DTT-treated panels, we provide packed RBCs which are negative for both E and K antigens if the patient lacks those antigens.

Hosokawa and colleagues[25] have described an alternative DTT method wherein a lower concentration of DTT (0.01 mol/L DTT) is used that disrupted the CD38 epitope

Table 3
Validation of DTT-treated RBCs for alloantibody detection at University of Chicago Medicine

Tested Antibodies			
RBC Antibody	**No. of Patient Samples**	**No. of Concordant Results**	**No. of Discrepant Results**
Anti-D	1	1	0
Anti-C	4	4	0
Anti-E	15	12	3
Anti-e	1	1	0
Anti-K	4	0 (expected with DTT effect)	N/A
Anti-Jka	2	2	0
Anti-Fya	2	2	0
Anti-M	1	1	0
Anti-S	4	4	0
Warm autoantibody	5	5	0

All clinically significant alloantibodies could be detected with DTT-treated RBCs confidently except for anti-K (as expected) as well as a subset of nascent (within 6 mo of initial detection) anti-E alloantibodies.

without complete destruction of the Kell antigen. This would allow use of DTT-treated panels for daratumumab-treated patients while retaining the ability to routinely rule out anti-K.

Enzyme treatment of reagent red cells for daratumumab mitigation has also been described, but has its own limitations and is unlikely to replace DTT.[14,22]

If patients are several weeks removed from daratumumab administration, it may be possible to rule-out all commonly clinically relevant alloantibodies by using a less sensitive technique for the antibody panels (eg, switching from a gel technique to a tube, or from a tube technique with polyethylene glycol to a tube technique with low ionic strength saline). This change may resolve interference without necessity for a DTT-treated panel in some patients.[29]

In summary, several modifications to pretransfusion testing have been described that can minimize daratumumab interference and ensure safe transfusion for patients receiving this mAb.[34] Each institution will have to perform their own cost analysis and decide which method is the most appropriate for their patient population.[35]

ANTI-CD47 AGENTS
CD47 Physiology

CD47, or integrin-associated protein, is a transmembrane glycoprotein molecule that is, found nearly ubiquitously on all tissues.

CD47 has several important cellular functions:

- Phagocytosis[36]
- Signaling after integrin binding to extracellular matrix[37,38]
- Apoptosis[39]
- Proliferation and angiogenesis[40]
- Adhesion and migration[41]

CD47 is a cellular defense that functions as a "do not eat me" signal.[42,43] CD47 inhibits cellular phagocytosis by engaging the macrophage SIRPα receptor. SIRPα belongs to the signal regulatory protein family and is expressed only on myeloid and neuronal cells. The binding of CD47 to macrophage SIRPα inhibits phagocytosis by activating macrophage immunoreceptor tyrosine-based inhibition motifs to recruit tyrosine phosphatases, SHP-1 and SHP-2, resulting in downstream negative regulation of macrophage effector functions.[44]

Interest in CD47 as a potential target for oncologic diseases lies in its overexpression on multiple tumors[36] and its interaction with SIRPα to prevent tumor cell phagocytosis. Targeting and neutralizing tumor cell CD47, in contrast, removes this inhibition of phagocytosis, facilitating the antitumor effect by macrophages.

CD47 is expressed on RBC as part of the band 3 complex[45] and expression of CD47 is decreased in Rh-null erythrocytes.[46] CD47 seems to play a role in red cell aging and survival in peripheral circulation: as red cells age and enter senescence, the amount of surface CD47 decreases.[47,48] This leads to increased RBC phagocytosis by splenic macrophages and clearance of aged RBCs.

Rather than the absolute amount of CD47 on the RBC membrane, other investigators have suggested a CD47 conformational change which converts the "do not eat me" signal into an "eat me" signal.[49–51]

Available Anti-CD47 Agents

No anti-CD47/SIRPα agents are currently FDA approved for treatment. However, there are multiple phase I trials and a phase II trial currently in progress involving various mAbs/recombinant proteins that target this pathway, either as monotherapy or in combination with an existing therapy (**Table 4** and clinicaltrials.gov).

Pharmacology of Anti-CD47 mAbs

Hu5F9-G4 (Forty-Seven, Inc., Menlo Park, CA) is a humanized mAb against CD47 with a human IgG4 Fc region. Studies of the pharmacokinetics of Hu5F9-G4 reveal similar properties as other IgG4 antibodies that are directed toward cell surface antigens: the half-life is reported to be approximately 14 days.[52]

Owing to the presence of CD47 antigens on normal tissues, anti-CD47 agents experience an "antigen sink" effect, which is saturated at doses of 10 mg/kg or greater. A maintenance dosing regimen of 30 mg/kg administered biweekly from cycle 2 onward results in serum concentrations of 200 μg/mL or greater, which has been correlated with complete saturation of CD47 on blood cells, as well as the efficacy of this therapy in preclinical trials.[52]

Effects on Pretransfusion Testing

Anti-CD47/SIRPα agents are relatively new, including some that are still in the recruitment phase of the clinical trial. Publication of trial results are still pending in many cases. For these reasons, definitive conclusions on the effects of anti-CD47/SIRPα agents on pretransfusion testing cannot be drawn for this class as a whole. Compounding this is, in our experience, the observation that different agents in this class demonstrate wide variability in their interference with pretransfusion testing. Therefore, additional published experience with these agents will be necessary before any broad statements can be made. We take this opportunity to urge pharmaceutical companies to share any and all knowledge of these agents' effects on pretransfusion testing with the broader transfusion community; such distribution of information will improve care for trial patients.

The most well-described effects of this mAb class are based on the anti-CD47 agent Hu5F9-G4 (**Table 5**). Hu5F9-G4 is an IgG4 monoclonal humanized antibody (mouse variable light chain attached to human IgG4 Fc region) targeted against CD47. The effects of Hu5F9-G4 on pretransfusion testing have been described in abstracts[53,54] and

Table 4
Anti-CD47 agents currently in clinical trials

Company and Name of Agent	Trial Identifier(s)	Agent Properties	Trial Indication(s)
Forty Seven, Inc. Hu5F9-G4	NCT02216409 NCT02678338 NCT02953509 NCT02953782 NCT03248479	IgG4 mAb; anti-CD47	AML, MDS, relapsed/refractory B-cell non-Hodgkin lymphoma, colorectal, and ovarian cancers
Celgene CC-90002	NCT02367196 NCT02641002	Humanized mAb; anti-CD47	AML, MDS, other hematologic neoplasms
Trillium Therapeutics TTI-621	NCT02663518 NCT02890368	Soluble recombinant fusion protein; N-terminal CD47 binding domain of human SIRPα with human IgG1 Fc domain	Hematologic malignancies, selected solid tumors
ALX Oncology ALX-148	NCT03013218	Fusion protein; 2 engineered high-affinity CD47 binding domains of SIRPα linked to an inactive human Fc region	Advanced solid tumors, non-Hodgkin lymphoma
Surface Oncology SRF231	NCT03512340	Human mAb; anti-CD47	Advanced solid cancers, hematologic cancers
Trillium Therapeutics TTI-622	NCT03530683	Soluble recombinant fusion protein; N-terminal CD47 binding domain of human SIRPα with human IgG4 Fc domain	Relapsed/refractory lymphoma or myeloma
Innovent Biologics IBI188	NCT03717103 NCT03763149	IgG4 mAb; Anti-CD47	Advanced malignancies

This list is not comprehensive, but representative of more recent and advanced clinical trials.
Abbreviations: AML, acute myeloid leukemia; MDS, myelodysplastic syndrome.

one recently published article and are corroborated by our experience at University of Chicago Medicine institutions (Zhen Mei, MD, unpublished data, 2018):

- Strong interference in ABO typing of non-blood group O patients (extra plasma reactivity in the back type)
- Pan-reactivity during antibody screening and identification
- Variably positive direct antiglobulin test
- Eluate with pan-agglutinin activity

It should be noted, however, that this pattern of interference does not reflect the entire anti-CD47/SIRPα class. Other anti-CD47 agents demonstrate less interference during plasma testing (Zhen Mei, MD, unpublished data, 2018):

- No interference in typing of patient blood
- Little to no extra reactivity during an antibody screen
- Strongly positive direct antiglobulin test
- Eluate demonstrates pan-agglutinin activity

Table 5
Representative pretransfusion testing results for one of the anti-CD47 agents

	Patient Results Before Anti-CD38 Therapy	Patient Results Post Anti-CD38 Therapy	Presence of Interference?
ABO/Rh typing	A+	Forward type: A+ Reverse type: O	Yes
Antibody Screen	Negative	Pan-reactive +	Yes
Autocontrol	Negative	Positive	Yes
Direct antiglobulin test	Negative	Negative/positive	Possible
Eluate	Not performed	Negative/pan-agglutinin	Possible

Noticeable interference is present during ABO/Rh typing for A, B, and AB patients. The antibody screen is always positive and can be resolved using a reagent that does not bind to IgG4 Fc regions.

The variability in the pattern of interference seen among different anti-CD47 agents may reflect variation in strength of the monoclonal affinity/avidity. Additional biochemical studies to elucidate this mechanism(s) are highly anticipated.

Resolution of Interference

At University of Chicago Medicine, the initial AHG reagent used during the observation of anti-CD47 mAb interferences was Ortho AHG (Ortho-Clinical Diagnostics, Raritan, NJ). This reagent functions to recognize and bind the Fc regions of any IgG antibodies that coat the surface of RBCs. However, there are 4 different IgG Fc regions, designated as IgG1, IgG2, IgG3, and IgG4.

When switching AHG reagents from Ortho AHG to Immucor AHG (Anti-IgG Murine Monoclonal [Green] Gamma-clone; Immucor, Peachtree Corners, GA), the pan-reactivity seen during antibody screen/identification in Hu5F9-G4–treated patients resolves, allowing underlying true alloantibodies to be detected.[53,54] Presumably, the Immucor AHG reagent does not recognize the IgG4 Fc region, and is thereby insensitive to the presence of Hu5F9-G4 coating the red cells.

SUMMARY

As mAb therapeutics become increasingly prevalent, the likelihood of samples from patients receiving these agents making their way to the blood bank increases as well. Without knowledge of the interference patterns seen with anti-CD38 and anti-CD47, or notification of patient treatment with these agents, elongated and burdensome laboratory workups are performed, resulting in a waste of reagent and labor resources, as well as delayed delivery of required blood products. Therefore, it becomes of paramount importance to improve communication between clinical care teams and blood banks. Efficacious patient care and timely blood product delivery are goals of every medical professional involved; therefore, both parties must be privy to the effects that new mAb agents may have on pretransfusion compatibility testing as well as knowledgeable as to the mAb received by a particular patient.

Clearer communication of use of anti-CD38 and anti-CD47 mAb will decrease the number of wasteful immunohematology workups performed on these samples. Communication from trial coordinators to the transfusion service is often excellent, but once mAb agents are FDA approved, the notification by ordering providers can become less optimal.

Overall the strategies to mitigate interference by these mAb agents can be divided into 3 different categories:

- Remove the presence of the target antigen on reagent RBC
- Neutralize the offending antibody
- Use different reagents that are less sensitive to the mAb effect

Although medical technologists are now increasingly able to recognize mAb interference patterns and obtain medication history from the electronic medical record,[55] the continued education of hematologists, blood bankers, and other laboratorians is necessary. Pharmaceutical companies involved in bringing these agents to market must play an important role in the dissemination of this knowledge. The transfusion community cannot wait for publication embargoes to lift before such knowledge can be disseminated; we must demand the ability to disseminate such important information as soon as we become aware of solutions. In partnership with our industry colleagues, we must either publish these solutions or seek alternative nonpublication dissemination mechanisms, if necessary.

ACKNOWLEDGMENTS

The authors would like to thank Marilyn Stewart MS Ed MT(ASCP)SBB for her work validating the DTT procedure for use in Daratumumab-treated patient samples at UCM. The authors would also like to thank Christine Howard-Menk, Dr. Jason Crane, and Dr. Mona Papari for data and helpful discussions of anti-CD47 cases.

REFERENCES

1. Köhler G, Milstein C. Continuous cultures of fused cells secreting antibody of predefined specificity. Nature 1975;256:495–7.
2. The Nobel Prize in Physiology or Medicine 1984 [press release]. Nobel Media AB 2018. 1984. Available at: https://www.nobelprize.org/prizes/medicine/1984/summary/. Accessed December 12, 2018.
3. Breedveld F. Therapeutic monoclonal antibodies. Lancet 2000;355:735–40.
4. Pierpont TM, Limper CB, Richards KL. Past, present, and future of rituximab-the world's first oncology monoclonal antibody therapy. Front Oncol 2018;8:163.
5. Singh S, Tank N, Dwiwedi P, et al. Monoclonal antibodies: a review. Curr Clin Pharmacol 2018;13:85–99.
6. Tang F, Malek E, Math S, et al. Interference of therapeutic monoclonal antibodies with routine serum protein electrophoresis and immunofixation in patients with myeloma: frequency and duration of detection of daratumumab and elotuzumab. Am J Clin Pathol 2018;150(2):121–9.
7. Keren DF. Therapeutic complications: a caveat for M-protein detection. J Appl Lab Med 2017;1(4):342–5.
8. Chen PP, Tormey CA, Eisenbarth SC, et al. False-positive light chain clonal restriction by flow cytometry in patients treated with alemtuzumab: potential pitfalls for the misdiagnosis of B-cell neoplasms. Am J Clin Pathol 2019;151(2):154–63.
9. Ferrero E, Malavasi F. The metamorphosis of a molecule: from soluble enzyme to the leukocyte receptor CD38. J Leukoc Biol 1999;65(2):151–61.
10. Mele S, Devereux S, Pepper AG. Calcium-RasGRP2-Rap1signaling mediates CD38- induced migration of chronic lymphocytic leukemia cells. Blood Adv 2018;2(13):1551–61.

11. Overdijk MB, Verploegen S, Bogels M, et al. Antibody-mediated phagocytosis contributes to the anti-tumor activity of the therapeutic antibody daratumumab in lymphoma and multiple myeloma. MAbs 2015;7:311–21.
12. Albeniz I, Demir O, Turker-Sener L, et al. Erythrocyte CD38 as a prognostic marker in cancer. Hematology 2007;12:409–14.
13. De Vooght KM, Oostendorp M, van Solinge WW. New mAb therapies in multiple myeloma: interference with blood transfusion compatibility testing. Curr Opin Hematol 2016;23(6):557–62.
14. Lancman G, Arinsburg S, Jhang J, et al. Blood transfusion management for patients treated with anti-CD38 monoclonal antibodies. Front Immunol 2018;9:2616.
15. Lokhorst H, Plesner T, Laubach J, et al. Targeting CD38 with daratumumab monotherapy in multiple myeloma. N Engl J Med 2015;373:1207–19.
16. van de Donk NWCJ, Richardson PG, Malavasi F. CD38 antibodies in multiple myeloma: back to the future. Blood 2018;131(1):13–29.
17. Clemens P, Yan X, Lokhorst H, et al. Pharmacokinetics of daratumumab following intravenous infusion in relapsed or refractory multiple myeloma after prior proteasome inhibitor and immunomodulatory drug treatment. Clin Pharmacokinet 2017; 58(8):915–24.
18. Jialal I, Pahwa R, Beck R, et al. Therapeutic monoclonal antibodies and the value of the free light chain assay in myeloma. Am J Clin Pathol 2018;150(5):468–9.
19. Oostendorp M, Lammerts van Bueren JJ, Doshi P, et al. When blood transfusion medicine becomes complicated due to interference by monoclonal antibody therapy. Transfusion 2015;55:1555–62.
20. Afifi S, Michael A, Lesokhin A. Immunotherapy: a new approach to treating multiple myeloma. Ann Pharmacother 2016;50(7):555–68.
21. Bub CB, Reis IND, Aravechia MG, et al. Transfusion management for patients taking an anti-CD38 monoclonal antibody. Rev Bras Hematol Hemoter 2018;40(1):25–9.
22. Carreño-Tarragona G, Cedena T, Montejano L, et al. Papain-treated panels are a simple method for the identification of alloantibodies in multiple myeloma patients treated with anti-CD38-based therapies. Transfus Med 2018.
23. Lin MH, Liu FY, Wang HM, et al. Interference of daratumumab with pretransfusion testing, mimicking a high-titer, low avidity like antibody. Asian J Transfus Sci 2017; 11(2):209–11.
24. Sullivan HC, Gerner-Smidt D, Nooka AK, et al. Daratumumab (anti-CD38) induces loss of CD38 on red blood cells. Blood 2017;129:3033–7.
25. Hosokawa M, Kashiwagi H, Nakayama K, et al. Distinct effects of daratumumab on indirect and direct antiglobulin tests: a new method employing 0.01 mol/L dithiothreitol for negating the daratumumab interference with preserving K antigenicity (Osaka method). Transfusion 2018;58(12):3003–13.
26. Deneys V, Thiry C, Frelik A, et al. Daratumumab: therapeutic asset, biological trap! Transfus Clin Biol 2018;25(1):2–7.
27. Quach H, Benson S, Haysom H, et al. Considerations for pre-transfusion immunohaematology testing in patients receiving the anti-CD38 monoclonal antibody daratumumab for the treatment of multiple myeloma. Intern Med J 2018;48(2):210–20.
28. Chapuy CI, Nicholson RT, Aguad MD, et al. Resolving the daratumumab interference with blood compatibility testing. Transfusion 2015;55:1545–54.
29. Lintel NJ, Brown DK, Schafer DT, et al. Use of standard laboratory methods to obviate routine dithiothreitol treatment of blood samples with daratumumab interference. Immunohematology 2017;33(1):22–6.
30. Chapuy CI, Aguad MD, Nicholson RT, et al, DARA-DTT Study Group* for the BEST Collaborative. International validation of a dithiothreitol (DTT)-based

method to resolve the daratumumab interference with blood compatibility testing. Transfusion 2016;56(12):2964–72.

31. Schmidt AE, Kirkley S, Patel N, et al. An alternative method to dithiothreitol treatment for antibody screening in patients receiving daratumumab. Transfusion 2015;55(9):2292–3.

32. Judd WJ, Johnson ST, Storry J. Judd's methods in immunohematology. 3rd edition. Bethesda (MD): American Association of Blood Banks; 2008.

33. Lorenzen H, Lone N, Nielsen M, et al. Thirty-three day storage of dithiothreitol-treated red blood cells used to eliminate daratumumab interference in serological testing. Vox Sang 2018;113(7):686–93.

34. Chari A, Arinsburg S, Jagannath S, et al. Blood transfusion management and transfusion-related outcomes in daratumumab-treated patients with relapsed or refractory multiple myeloma. Clin Lymphoma Myeloma Leuk 2018;18(1):44–51.

35. Anani WQ, Marchan MG, Bensing KM, et al. Practical approaches and costs for provisioning safe transfusions during anti-CD38 therapy. Transfusion 2017;57(6): 1470–9.

36. Chao MP, Weissman IL, Majeti R. The CD47-SIRPα pathway in cancer immune evasion and potential therapeutic implications. Curr Opin Immunol 2012;24(2): 225–32.

37. Oldenborg PA, Zheleznyak A, Fang YF, et al. Role of CD47 as a marker of self on red blood cells. Science 2000;288(5473):2051–4.

38. Russ A, Hua A, Montfort W, et al. Blocking "don't eat me" signal of CD47-SIRPα in hematological malignancies, an in-depth review. Blood Rev 2018;32(6):480–9.

39. Leclair P, Liu CC, Monajemi M, et al. CD47-ligation induced cell death in T-acute lymphoblastic leukemia. Cell Death Dis 2018;9(5):544.

40. Kaur S, Chang T, Singh SP, et al. CD47 signaling regulates the immunosuppressive activity of VEGF in T cells. J Immunol 2014;193(8):3914–24.

41. Talme T, Bergdahl E, Sundqvist KG. Regulation of T-lymphocyte motility, adhesion and de-adhesion by a cell surface mechanism directed by low density lipoprotein receptor-related protein 1 and endogenous thrombospondin-1. Immunology 2014;142(2):176–92.

42. van den Berg TK, van Bruggen R. Loss of CD47 makes dendritic cells see red. Immunity 2015;43(4):622–4.

43. Olsson M, Nilsson A, Oldenborg PA. Dose-dependent inhibitory effect of CD47 in macrophage uptake of IgG-opsonized murine erythrocytes. Biochem Biophys Res Commun 2007;352(1):193–7.

44. Ho CC, Guo N, Sockolosky JT, et al. "Velcro" engineering of high affinity CD47 ectodomain as signal regulatory protein α (SIRPα) antagonists that enhance antibody-dependent cellular phagocytosis. J Biol Chem 2015;290(20):12650–63.

45. Oldenborg PA. Role of CD47 in erythroid cells and in autoimmunity. Leuk Lymphoma 2004;45(7):1319–27.

46. Lindberg FP, Lublin DM, Telen MJ, et al. Rh-related antigen CD47 is the signal-transducer integrin-associated protein. J Biol Chem 1994;269:1567–70.

47. Khandelwal S, van Rooijen N, Saxena RK. Reduced expression of CD47 during murine red blood cell (RBC) senescence and its role in RBC clearance from the circulation. Transfusion 2007;47(9):1725–32.

48. Olsson M, Oldenborg PA. CD47 on experimentally senescent murine RBCs inhibits phagocytosis following Fcgamma receptor-mediated but not scavenger receptor-mediated recognition by macrophages. Blood 2008;112(10):4259–67.

49. van Bruggen R. CD47 functions as a removal marker on aged erythrocytes. ISBT Sci Ser 2013;8:153–6.

50. Burger P, de Korte D, van den Berg TK, et al. CD47 in erythrocyte ageing and clearance - the Dutch point of view. Transfus Med Hemother 2012;39(5):348–52.
51. Burger P, Hilarius-Stokman P, de Korte D, et al. CD47 functions as a molecular switch for erythrocyte phagocytosis. Blood 2012;119(23):5512–21.
52. Agoram B, Wang B, Sikic B. Pharmacokinetics of Hu5F9-G4, a first-in-class anti-CD47 antibody, in patients with solid tumors and lymphomas. J Clin Oncol 2018; 36(15):2525. Abstract.
53. Velliquette R, Aeschlimann J, Kirkegaard J, et al. Monoclonal anti-CD47 interference in red cell and platelet testing. Transfusion 2019;59(2):730–7.
54. Nedelcu E, Hall C, Stoner A, et al. Interference of Anti-CD47 Therapy with Blood Bank Testing. Poster presented at: AABB 2017 Annual Meeting. San Diego, CA, October 7–10.
55. Anani WQ, Duffer K, Kaufman RM, et al. How do I work up pretransfusion samples containing anti-CD38? Transfusion 2017;57(6):1337–42.

Impact of Genotyping on Selection of Red Blood Cell Donors for Transfusion

Ronald Jackups Jr, MD, PhD

KEYWORDS

- RBC antigen genotyping • RBC antigen serology • RBC antigen phenotype
- RBC donor selection

KEY POINTS

- Serology is the primary method of red blood cell (RBC) antigen phenotyping for determining transfusion compatibility, but it suffers from several sources of interference and low throughput.
- High-throughput genotyping offers advantages compared with serology for RBC antigen phenotyping in several patient populations in hematology and oncology.
- Genotyping has limitations, including genotype-phenotype discrepancies and need for high-complexity testing.
- At present, genotyping should be used as an adjunct to serology for RBC antigen phenotyping in complex cases, but it may supplant serology in the future as technology advances.

INTRODUCTION

Red blood cells (RBCs) express many proteins and glycoproteins on their cell surfaces, which perform various functions, including structural support, enzymatic reactions, and transport of molecules.[1] Polymorphisms in the genes encoding these proteins, or encoding enzymes that alter the structure of glycoproteins, result in the formation of antigens that may complicate blood compatibility testing, because of the risk of alloimmunization. There are more than 300 such antigens, although only 20 to 30 antigens are evaluated in routine clinical testing.[2]

Blood compatibility testing, whose purpose is to identify blood components safe for transfusion to particular patients, relies primarily on the identification of clinically

Disclosure: The author received funding from an unrestricted educational grant provided to Wiley by Bio-Rad.

Department of Pathology & Immunology, Washington University School of Medicine, 660 South Euclid Avenue #8118, St Louis, MO 63110, USA

E-mail address: rjackups@wustl.edu

significant antibodies to RBC antigens. Antigen phenotyping is an essential complement to this process, because it can confirm whether antibodies are allogeneic or autologous in origin. However, phenotyping may serve additional roles in hematology and oncology patients, including prophylaxis against alloimmunization, identification of rare antigen variants that may complicate compatibility testing, screening for engraftment and complications in ABO-nonidentical bone marrow and organ transplants, and resolution of difficult blood compatibility evaluations complicated by autoantibodies or certain medications, such as daratumumab.

For nearly a century, the primary laboratory methods for RBC antigen phenotyping have been serologic, relying on direct identification of antibody-antigen reactions. Although this is effective in most routine cases, recent studies have shown that certain populations, including those with hematologic conditions, are at high risk of developing antibodies, even when cleared by serologic compatibility testing.[3–5] In addition, technological advances have shown the promise of genotyping as an effective complement or even replacement to serology. This article describes the differences between phenotyping strategies, the current indications for genotyping in the hematology/oncology population, and the challenges and future directions of this technology.

SEROLOGIC PHENOTYPING FOR RED BLOOD CELL ANTIGENS

Before the use of genotyping technology to identify RBC antigens, most phenotyping was performed by serologic methods. This approach involved the use of reagent antibodies with known specificities, which would be incubated with patient or donor RBCs of unknown antigen status, with or without anti–human globulin (Coombs reagent). Visible agglutination would indicate that the antigen corresponding to the reagent antibody was present on the RBC surface. This methodology serves 2 major purposes. First, phenotyping of a patient's RBCs confirms whether an antibody in the patient's blood was caused by alloimmunization (if the patient's RBCs tested negative for the corresponding antigen) or by an autoimmune process (if the patient's RBCs tested positive for the antigen); this distinction is critical for determining both the cause of the patient's antibody and the safe selection of blood products for transfusion. Second, phenotyping of an RBC-containing blood product allows identification of antigen-negative units safe to transfuse to a patient with a known alloantibody.

Serology is considered the gold standard for RBC antigen phenotyping in most patients, because it confirms the active expression of the antigen of interest.[2] This method overcomes a major limitation of genetic testing, which primarily can only identify the genes encoding the antigens, rather than the expression patterns themselves. However, serologic phenotyping suffers from several limitations and confounding factors that may make the method unsuitable for specific patients, particularly those with hematologic and oncologic disease (**Table 1**). Serologic testing requires several manual steps, and only 1 antigen can be evaluated per test, limiting the throughput. Testing for rarely encountered antigens may be very expensive or even unavailable at most sites, because of the difficulty of obtaining reagent antibodies with rare specificities. False-negative results may occur when antigens are weakly expressed, or unexpected variant antigens are present that may not be detected by the reagent antibody. In addition, false-positive results may occur in patients who express variant antigens not intended to be identified by the reagent antibody, were recently transfused with allogeneic blood, or who received treatment with specific monoclonal antibodies (eg, daratumumab, anti–cluster of differentiation [CD] 47).[6,7]

Table 1	
Limitations of serologic and genetic testing for red blood cell antigen phenotyping	
Serologic Testing	**Genotyping**
Low throughput (1 antigen per test)	Requires specialized equipment and technologists trained in molecular testing
Typing reagents unavailable and/or not FDA approved for rarely tested antigens	FDA approval limited to antigen variants encoded by single nucleotide polymorphisms
False-positives/negatives caused by variant alleles	Long turnaround time in most clinical situations
Interference caused by prior transfusion, autoantibodies, and monoclonal antibody therapies (anti-CD38 and anti-CD47)	Can only predict, rather than verify, antigen expression on RBC surface in most cases

Abbreviations: CD, cluster of differentiation; FDA, US Food and Drug Administration.

Serologic phenotyping continues to serve an essential role in facilitating the identification of compatible blood for patients with 1 or a few common RBC antibodies (eg, Rh, Kell, Duffy). However, more complicated clinical situations call for high-throughput genetic testing, as described later.

GENOTYPING FOR RED BLOOD CELL ANTIGENS

Genotyping for RBC antigens involves the identification of polymorphisms that differentiate antigens of clinical significance. The most commonly encountered polymorphisms are caused by single base pair changes, which can be detected by a variety of testing methods. However, more complicated polymorphisms exist and are fairly common in the 2 most clinically significant blood groups, ABO and Rh, requiring more complex testing methods.[3]

A US Food and Drug Administration (FDA)–approved technology for RBC antigen detection by genotyping involves the use of a multiplexed polymerase chain reaction (PCR) and hybridization-based assay.[8,9] Briefly, DNA is extracted from the patient's specimen, subjected to multiplexed PCR of the regions of interest, and hybridized onto oligonucleotide probes for common antigen alleles. If a sequence corresponding with a particular antigen is present, it is detected by the use of fluorophores.[10,11] Because the method is multiplexed, multiple antigens (>30) can be detected at the same time in a high-throughput assay.

At present, FDA approval extends only to 2 assays that cover ~30 to 40 of the most commonly evaluated RBC antigens in routine blood banking, in such blood groups as Rh, Kell, Duffy, Kidd, and MNS.[8,9] This technology has been extended to other menus of antigens, particularly to less common variant antigens in the Rh system, although it is limited to only those antigens that can be detected reliably by single nucleotide polymorphisms. Next-generation sequencing (NGS) is a promising alternative that is under active investigation by multiple laboratories, although its use in clinical care is currently limited.[3,12,13] NGS may surpass older technologies, because of its higher throughput and potential to identify more complicated polymorphisms.[3]

Although genotyping offers distinct advantages compared with serologic methods for identifying RBC antigens, it also carries unique limitations (see **Table 1**). The testing is far more complex than serology, requiring both expensive equipment and specialized technologists to perform, and thus it is primarily limited to reference laboratories. For this reason, the turnaround time is often too long to facilitate urgent clinical questions. A less well-understood limitation is that, unlike serology, genotyping does not directly detect expression of an antigen on the RBC surface; expression must be inferred based on the presence of specific DNA patterns.[3] Although genotype-phenotype correlation is highly accurate in most routine cases, the presence of unde-tected polymorphisms in regulatory domains can lead to incorrect calls. The most common example is a mutation in an erythroid-specific promoter (GATA box) for the gene encoding Duffy alleles. Genetically, the allele may appear to be a standard Fy^b allele, but, in actuality, the allele does not express Fy^b on the RBC surface, and in the homozygous state leads to null expression of all Duffy antigens on RBCs.[1] This Duffy-null expression pattern is seen in approximately two-thirds of individuals of Af-rican descent, so any testing method must account for it. Fortunately, the promoter mutation is also caused by a single nucleotide change, so it is routinely included in currently offered genetic panels.[10]

Although genotype-phenotype correlation poses some challenges for genotyping, it can sometimes reveal serologic typing errors. Because serologic phenotyping is a more manual process, clerical or other preanalytical errors may be detected by genetic methods.[14] More importantly, unexpected variant alleles may be present that are iden-tified by serologic reagents as common alleles but are different enough at the molecular level to induce alloimmunization when a patient with such a variant allele is transfused with blood expressing the common allele. Such variants are sometimes called partial alleles, and their presence is more common in certain blood groups (especially Rh) and in certain patient populations.[2] Hundreds of such variant alleles have been identi-fied, and the identification of such alleles is an area of active research.[1,15]

Overall, serologic and genetic methods for RBC antigen phenotyping offer different advantages and limitations in current blood banking processes and transfusion deci-sions, and they will likely remain competing but complementary techniques for some time (see **Table 1**). Understanding these differences is critical to selecting the appro-priate method for different patient scenarios in hematology and oncology.

INDICATIONS FOR RED BLOOD CELL ANTIGEN GENOTYPING IN HEMATOLOGY AND ONCOLOGY

Transfusion is a common procedure in patients with hematologic or oncologic dis-ease, and transfusion decisions in these patients are often more complicated than in other specialties. Although genotyping is potentially useful for any patient at risk of requiring transfusion, there are several groups in which genotyping has shown clin-ical utility (**Box 1**). These groups can largely be characterized by 2 fundamental indi-cations: patients for whom serologic testing would be inaccurate, and patients with complex transfusion needs that would be best served by high-throughput testing.

Box 1
Indications for red blood cell antigen genotyping in hematology and oncology patients

- Situations in which serologic testing is inaccurate
  - Patients who have been recently transfused
  - Patients with RBC autoantibodies or complex alloantibody profiles
  - Patients receiving monoclonal antibody (anti-CD38 or anti-CD47) therapy
  - Patients with weakly reactive Rh testing by serology

- Patients with complex transfusion needs
  - Patients with sickle cell disease receiving chronic transfusion therapy
  - Patients with sickle cell disease receiving hematopoietic stem cell transplant
  - Patients with malignancies receiving hematopoietic stem cell transplant
  - Patients with current or prior history of RBC alloimmunization

---

Recently Transfused Patients

Transfused RBCs may remain in a patient's bloodstream for 2 to 3 months.[16] Because serologic testing is based on the identification of antigens on RBCs, antigen expression on transfused RBCs may lead to a false prediction that those antigens are native to the patient. If a recent transfusion is implicated in a hemolytic transfusion reaction, the resulting antibody may be mistakenly characterized as an autoantibody. For these reasons, it is critical to interpret serologic testing in the context of the patient's transfusion history and to alert the blood bank of such history in the case of discrepant testing. Genotyping relies on a source of DNA, such as the patient's white blood cells, rather than RBCs, and therefore does not suffer the same interference. In most cases, serologic techniques are sufficient to resolve the discrepancies, but, in the case of patients transfused multiple units over time, genetic testing may be preferred.

Patients with Autoantibodies or Complicated Alloantibodies

Most autoantibodies encountered in transfusion practice are panreactive, meaning that they react with nearly every donor RBC unit tested. It is therefore standard practice, in situations in which autoimmune hemolytic anemia is life threatening, to provide crossmatch-incompatible RBCs for transfusion, because no available blood will be compatible in vitro.[17] Before releasing incompatible units, blood banks should perform additional testing to rule out the presence of alloantibodies obscured by the autoantibody, but this testing is labor intensive and not always successful in ruling out clinically significant alloantibodies. In these situations, genotyping provides an effective method to predict the patient's RBC antigen phenotype, and, when there is uncertainty about the presence of alloantibodies, RBC units that are negative for the antigens that the patient does not express can be used as an additional safety measure.

Likewise, there are situations in which patient specimens with multiple alloantibodies or an alloantibody to a high-frequency antigen may lead to uncertainty in compatibility testing. Some of these alloantibodies, such as high-titer, low-avidity–like antibodies, are not clinically significant but present unavoidable interference in ruling out clinically significant alloantibodies.[2,17] As with autoantibodies, the use of genotyping may allow additional safety in the identification of appropriate blood for transfusion.

Patients on Monoclonal Antibody Therapy that Interferes with Blood Bank Testing

Daratumumab, an anti-CD38 monoclonal antibody therapy, was approved by the FDA for treatment of multiple myeloma.[18] Because CD38 is expressed on RBCs, compatibility testing on patients currently taking daratumumab will suffer from interference caused by the drug being bound on the patients' RBCs.[6] Although methods do exist to resolve this interference, those that are available to most blood banks introduce other complications. The most common method is the use of dithiothreitol (DTT), a reducing agent that removes reactivity to CD38 on RBCs.[6] However, DTT also eliminates expression of other RBC antigens, most notably those in the Kell blood group system, leaving standard compatibility testing incomplete.[1] One solution is to perform DTT treatment on every sample throughout the patient's treatment and provide RBC units negative for K (the most common Kell antigen associated with alloimmunization) when needed. However, another attractive option would be to use genotyping to determine which of the clinically significant RBC antigens the patient is negative for, then select blood products negative for those antigens throughout treatment. Although a full serologic phenotype could be performed before taking the drug, genotyping offers higher throughput and is the only option if the patient has already started the medication, which is when the interference is usually first identified.

Hu5F9-G4, a monoclonal antibody designed to block CD47, is under active clinical trials for the treatment of both hematologic malignancies and solid tumors.[19] However, this drug interferes with transfusion compatibility testing in a similar way as anti-CD38 antibodies, but this interference cannot be removed with compounds such as DTT.[7] Although some techniques were identified as having the potential to resolve the interference, it is not clear how they affect identification of clinically significant antibodies.[7] This uncertainty makes an even stronger case than anti-CD38 for the utility of RBC antigen genotyping to improve the safety of blood product selection.

For more detailed information about the impact of monoclonal antibody therapy on serologic blood bank testing, please see Drs Zhen Mei and Geoffrey D. Wool's article, "Impact of Novel Monoclonal Antibody Therapeutics on Blood Bank Pretransfusion Testing," in this issue.

Patients with Current or Previous History of Antibodies

Although the genetic and immunologic mechanisms are not entirely clear, it is well known that patients who have already made RBC alloantibodies are at a higher risk than the general population of making additional alloantibodies; such patients are sometimes called responders.[20,21] This risk is even higher in patients with sickle cell disease.[5] In practice, patients without antibodies are transfused blood that is proactively matched for ABO and RhD antigens only, because ABO antibodies are preformed in infancy, and RhD is the most immunogenic of the remaining common blood group antigens.[2] However, in patients who have already shown that they are responders, some facilities go to extra lengths to protect the patients from alloimmunization against additional antigens. This practice of extended matching involves phenotyping the patient's RBC antigens, then selecting blood products that are negative for the antigens that the patient lacks.[3,22] The most immunogenic antigens, particularly in the Rh and Kell systems, are given priority, but other clinically significant antigens, such as those in the Duffy and Kidd groups, may be included. Serologic phenotyping may facilitate this process for a limited number of antigens, such as C, E, and K, but, as the panel becomes larger, the use of single-antigen typing reagents becomes less cost-effective, particularly at centers where reagents for rarely tested antigens are not routinely available. Genotyping with a high-throughput assay then becomes an optimal method to determine status for many antigens at once.

At centers that may care for complex patients with positive antibody histories, especially those with a large sickle cell population, use of such extended matching protocols requires an inventory of RBC products typed for the same antigens as those tested in patients.[22] Therefore, donors are often genotyped by the same methods. At centers that both treat patients and collect blood products for general use, repeat donors can be tested, and those with rare phenotypes can be encouraged to donate more often. At centers that acquire products from external sources, such as large regional or national blood suppliers, this option is more limited. Samples from blood products delivered to the center could be genotyped, but with the increasing use of leukoreduced blood in the United States,[23] more specialized and non–FDA-approved assays would have to be used.[5]

Patients with Sickle Cell Disease Receiving Chronic Transfusion Therapy

Patients with sickle cell disease who have received chronic transfusion therapy have considerably higher rates of alloimmunization (~30% or more) than the general population,[24] and those who develop antibodies are more likely to make more.[5] Therefore, patients on chronic transfusion therapy are usually provided extended antigen matching, as described earlier. Although the most cited matching strategy only extends to the C, E, and K antigens, some institutions that specialize in sickle cell disease have chosen to match beyond those antigens (eg to include Duffy and Kidd).[5,25,26]

Even more challenging is the higher prevalence of variant alleles in patients of African descent, most notably in the Rh system (RHD and RHCE genes).[1] Such alleles may serologically type as a common antigen, but still carry the risk of alloimmunization; patients who are transfused units appropriately matched for Rh may still have breakthrough alloimmunization.[4] These partial alleles cannot be accounted for by routine serologic testing, and therefore the only way to identify them is by genotyping.[27] However, even with the use of genotyping, identifying these patients may be challenging, because more and more variants alleles are identified and reported in the literature.[3,15] In addition, such variant alleles may be so rare that it becomes difficult to identify compatible donors and maintain adequate inventory to support chronic transfusion therapy.[3] Prophylactic genotyping for Rh variants, before the patient has made antibodies, presents an additional ethical concern: would it be more appropriate to use rare donor units to prevent alloimmunization in these patients or to preserve such units for those who have already made antibodies? The implications of this dilemma are discussed in more detail later.

In addition to facilitating extended matching, genotype prediction of RBC antigen phenotype in patients with sickle cell disease provides one more notable advantage to hematologists: if the patient is identified to be negative for a high-prevalence antigen, or to carry homozygous or compound heterozygous variant Rh alleles, that status may serve as an additional consideration for patients with severe disease under consideration for hematopoietic stem cell transplant (HSCT).[28] Although it may pose difficulty for matching blood products in the peritransplant phase, it may make chronic transfusion therapy, which requires many more blood transfusions over the patient's lifetime, inaccessible.

Patients with Sickle Cell Disease Receiving Hematopoietic Stem Cell Transplant

HSCT is an increasingly popular treatment of patients with severe complications of sickle cell disease.[29] Because such patients have often received chronic transfusion therapy, they have the same history and risks of alloimmunization as described earlier, but their course is further complicated by the donor's RBC antigen status. It is therefore advisable to phenotype both the patient and potential donors in order to make transfusion decisions proactively.[30]

Conditioning for HSCT to treat sickle cell disease is often nonmyeloablative, resulting in mixed lymphocyte chimerism.[31] For this reason, it cannot be reliably predicted whether the patient's previous alloantibodies will persist after transplant, and moreover whether the patient retains the higher of risk of alloimmunization identified in sickle cell disease. The decision of whether to honor extended prophylactic matching protocols or difficult matching for rare alleles must therefore be individualized. In any event, high-throughput genotyping provides the most information for the clinical team to make well-directed decisions.

Patients with Malignancies Receiving Allogeneic Hematopoietic Stem Cell Transplant

RBC alloimmunization is also a risk for patients with malignancies receiving HSCT, although this risk is not as significant as in sickle cell disease. It is estimated that 2% to 9% of patients develop RBC alloantibodies following transplant.[32,33] There may be a role for matching HSCT donor and recipient for non-ABO RBC antigens, although current limited evidence in Rh-mismatched and Kell-mismatched pairs does not show a significant detrimental effect on engraftment.[33]

Regardless, high-throughput RBC antigen phenotyping may aid in selection of both donors and blood products, as discussed earlier for sickle cell disease.[30] If phenotyping of the recipient is required following transplant, the recipient's original phenotype can be obtained by genotyping of a buccal specimen to avoid interference by the donor's engrafted blood cells.

Patients with Weakly Reacting RhD Serologic Testing

Testing for the presence of RhD antigen is a required component of the standard type and screen. Typically, RhD-positive specimens react very strongly with anti-D reagent, resulting in a large visible agglutinate (graded as 4+). On rare occasions, usually in patients who have never been tested, a weakly positive reaction may occur, in which small but barely visible agglutinates may be seen (graded as 2+ or lower). If this weak reaction cannot be explained by recent transfusion with D-negative RBCs, the presence of an Rh variant allele may be suspected, particularly in patients of African descent, in whom Rh variants are more common. In such situations, it is advisable to perform genotyping to identify Rh variants, even before the patient has made an alloantibody, to prevent alloimmunization.[34,35] Testing for variants in both the RHD and RHCE genes may be considered, particularly in patients who are likely to receive multiple transfusions, such as those with sickle cell disease. Before testing can be completed, RhD-negative RBC units should be selected for transfusion. If genotyping does reveal the presence of partial antigens that confer a risk of alloimmunization, the patient should be made aware, in order to relay this information at future hospital visits, to aid clinical teams in providing Rh-negative RBCs.

Pregnant Women with Pregnancies at Risk of Hemolytic Disease of the Newborn

Note that genotyping is a common method for RBC antigen identification in fetuses at risk of hemolytic disease of the newborn, and for women with weakly reactive RhD testing at time of delivery, to inform dosing of Rh immune globulin. However, because these patients are encountered primarily in obstetrics, these clinical indications are not discussed further but are available in other literature.[3,35]

CHALLENGES AND FUTURE DIRECTIONS FOR RED BLOOD CELL ANTIGEN PHENOTYPING AND MATCHING

As the use of genotyping for RBC antigen determination increases, and the technology behind it becomes more accurate and cost-effective,[3,36] several opportunities and challenges will present themselves in the clinical care of hematology and oncology patients, as well as all patients who may need transfusion and individuals who donate blood.

First, discrepancies in genotype-phenotype correlation will need to be identified and resolved in order to improve the accuracy of genotyping to the degree that it may be used as the test of record for all testing indications. Assays based on single nucleotide polymorphisms are inadequate to detect all clinically significant polymorphisms, but NGS shows promise in bridging the gap. The greatest difficulties lie in verifying the cause of genotype-phenotype discrepancies, because they may occur in very small populations worldwide, and in predicting possible discrepancies de novo based on gene networks.

Second, genetic phenotypes of donors must be made available on a wider scale than single regional blood centers. This availability will facilitate matching of blood products for patients with rare antigen phenotypes or complex serologic profiles.[37] The use of such databases has been shown to be feasible on a regional level.[38] However, care must be taken to ensure both the security of donors' protected health information and the equitable use of donor recruitment strategies to satisfy the needs of relevant patient populations.

Finally, as genotype information becomes more readily available and accurate, effective matching strategies must be developed to minimize the risk of clinically significant antigen mismatches and ensure the durability of the national blood supply. Such a balance is not simple, because it must account for the immunogenicity of each antigen and the potential for a patient to be a responder in order to determine the value of prophylactic matching, as opposed to the current reactive process of only matching after a patient has created an antibody. A well-designed bioinformatic algorithm could attain this goal, but it would still need to be tempered by the ethics of maintaining an inventory large enough to support high-risk patients who have made antibodies.

In summary, genotyping technology offers advantages compared with serologic techniques for determining the RBC antigen phenotypes of both donors and patients with hematologic and oncologic disease, but additional improvements in technology and practical considerations are needed before it can supplant serology as the gold standard. In the meantime, its value in specific patient populations, such as patients with RBC antibodies, sickle cell disease, and certain hematologic malignancies, has already been clearly demonstrated.

ACKNOWLEDGMENTS

The author would like to thank Chang Liu, MD, PhD, and Suzanne Thibodeaux, MD, PhD, for helpful discussions.

REFERENCES

1. Reid ME, Lomas-Francis C, Olsson ML, editors. The blood group antigen factsbook. 3rd edition. Waltham (MA): Elsevier; 2012.
2. Fung MK, Eder AF, Spitalnik SL, et al, editors. Technical manual. 19th edition. Bethesda (MD): AABB; 2017.
3. Westhoff CM. Blood group genotyping. Blood 2019. https://doi.org/10.1192/blood-2018-11-833954.
4. Chou ST, Jackson T, Vege S, et al. High prevalence of red blood cell alloimmunization in sickle cell disease despite transfusion from Rh-matched minority donors. Blood 2013;122:1062–71.
5. Yee MEM, Josephson CD, Winkler AM, et al. Red blood cell minor antigen mismatches during chronic transfusion therapy for sickle cell anemia. Transfusion 2017;57:2738–46.
6. Chapuy CI, Nicholson RT, Aguad MD, et al. Resolving the daratumumab interference with blood compatibility testing. Transfusion 2015;55:1545–54.
7. Velliquette RW, Aeschlimann J, Kirkegaard J, et al. Monoclonal anti-CD47 interference in red cell and platelet testing. Transfusion 2019;59:730–7.
8. May 21, 2014 Approval letter – Immucor PreciseType. Available at: https://www.fda.gov/BiologicsBloodVaccines/BloodBloodProducts/ApprovedProducts/PremarketApprovalsPMAs/ucm399034.htm. Accessed April 15, 2019.
9. October 11, 2018 Approval letter – Grifols ID CORE XT. Available at: https://www.fda.gov/BiologicsBloodVaccines/BloodBloodProducts/ApprovedProducts/PremarketApprovalsPMAs/ucm623204.htm. Accessed April 17, 2019.

10. Wilkinson DS. Clinical utility of genotyping human erythrocyte antigens. Lab Med 2016;47:e28–31.

11. Lopez M, Apraiz I, Rubia M, et al. Performance evaluation study of ID CORE XT, a high throughput blood group genotyping platform. Blood Transfus 2018;16: 193–9.

12. Lane WJ, Westhoff CM, Gleadall NS, et al. Automated typing of red blood cell and platelet antigens: a whole-genome sequencing study. Lancet Hematol 2018;5: e241–51.

13. Fichou Y, Audrezet MP, Gueguen P, et al. Next-generation sequencing is a credible strategy for blood group genotyping. Br J Haematol 2014;167:554–62.

14. Casas J, Friedman DF, Jackson T, et al. Changing practice: red blood cell typing by molecular methods for patients with sickle cell disease. Transfusion 2015;55: 1388–93.

15. Vege S, Westhoff CM. Molecular characterization of GYPB and RH in donors in the American Rare Donor Program. Immunohematology 2006;22:143–7.

16. Klein HG, Anstee DJ. The transfusion of red cells. In: Klein HG, Anstee DJ, editors. Mollison's blood transfusion in clinical medicine. Malden (MA): Blackwell Publishing; 2005. p. 352–63.

17. Lee E, Redman M, Burgess G, et al. Do patients with autoantibodies or clinically insignificant alloantibodies require an indirect antiglobulin test crossmatch? Transfusion 2007;47:1290–5.

18. Daratumumab (DARZALEX). Available at: https://www.fda.gov/drugs/information ondrugs/approveddrugs/ucm530249.htm. Accessed April 15, 2019.

19. Clinical Trials Using Anti-CD47 Monoclonal Antibody Hu5F9-G4. Available at: https://www.cancer.gov/about-cancer/treatment/clinical-trials/intervention/anti-cd47-monoclonal-antibody-hu5f9-g4. Accessed April 15, 2019.

20. Higgins JM, Sloan SR. Stochastic modeling of human RBC alloimmunization: evidence for a distinct population of immunologic responders. Blood 2008;112: 2546–53.

21. Schonewille H, van de Watering LMG, Brand A. Additional red blood cell alloantibodies after blood transfusions in a nonhematologic alloimmunized patient cohort: is it time to take precautionary measures? Transfusion 2006;46:630–5.

22. Klapper E, Zhang Y, Figueroa P, et al. Toward extended phenotype matching: a new operational paradigm for the transfusion service. Transfusion 2010;50: 536–46.

23. National Blood Collection & Utilization Survey. Available at: https://www.hhs.gov/ohaidp/initiatives/blood-tissue-safety/initiatives/national-blood-collection-and-utilization-survey/index.html. Accessed April 15, 2019.

24. Matteocci A, Pierelli L. Red blood cell alloimmunization in sickle cell disease and in thalassemia: current status, future perspectives and potential role of molecular typing. Vox Sang 2014;106:197–208.

25. Rees DC, Robinson S, Howard J. How I manage red cell transfusions in patients with sickle cell disease. Br J Hematol 2018;180:607–17.

26. Fichou Y, Mariez M, Le Marechal C, et al. The experience of extended blood group genotyping by next-generation sequencing (NGS): investigation of patients with sickle-cell disease. Vox Sang 2016;111:418–24.

27. Flegel WA, von Zabern I, Wagner FF. Six years' experience performing RHD genotyping to confirm D- red blood cell units in Germany for preventing anti-D immunizations. Transfusion 2009;49:465–71.

28. Fasano RM, Monaco A, Meier ER, et al. RH genotyping in a sickle cell disease patient contributing to hematopoietic stem cell transplantation donor selection and management. Blood 2010;116:2836–8.
29. Hulbert ML, Shenoy S. Hematopoietic stem cell transplantation for sickle cell disease: progress and challenges. Pediatr Blood Cancer 2018;65:e27263.
30. Allen ES, Nelson RC, Flegel WA. How we evaluate red blood cell compatibility and transfusion support for patients with sickle cell disease undergoing hematopoietic progenitor cell transplantation. Transfusion 2018;58:2483–9.
31. Hsieh MM, Fitzhugh CD, Weitzel RP. Nonmyeloablative HLA-matched sibling allogeneic hematopoietic stem cell transplantation for severe sickle cell phenotype. JAMA 2014;312:48–56.
32. Booth GS, Gehrie EA, Savani BN. Minor RBC Ab and allo-SCT. Bone Marrow Transplant 2014;49:456–7.
33. Rowley SD, Donato ML, Bhattacharyya P, et al. Red blood cell-incompatible allogeneic hematopoietic progenitor cell transplantation. Bone Marrow Transplant 2011;46:1167–85.
34. Sandler SG, Chen LN, Flegel WA. Serological weak D phenotypes: a review and guidance for interpreting the RhD blood type using the RHD genotype. Br J Hematol 2017;179:10–9.
35. Kacker S, Vassallo R, Keller MA, et al. Financial implications of RHD genotyping of pregnant women with a serologic weak D phenotype. Transfusion 2015;55:2095–103.
36. Kacker S, Ness PM, Savage WJ, et al. Cost-effectiveness of prospective red blood cell antigen matching to prevent alloimmunization among sickle cell patients. Transfusion 2014;54:86–97.
37. Klein HG, Flegel WA, Natanson C. Red blood cell transfusion: precision vs. imprecision medicine. JAMA 2015;314:1557–8.
38. Flegel WA, Gottschall JL, Denomme GA. Integration of red cell genotyping into the blood supply chain: a population-based study. Lancet Hematol 2015;2:e282–8.

Advances in T-cell Immunotherapies

David F. Stroncek, MD*, Opal Reddy, MD, Steven Highfill, PhD,
Sandhya R. Panch, MD

KEYWORDS

- Cell processing • Cancer immunotherapy • Donor lymphocyte infusions
- Virus-specific T cells • Chimeric antigen receptor T cells
- Tumor-infiltrating lymphocytes

KEY POINTS

- T-cell immunotherapies have become an important cancer therapy.
- Chimeric antigen receptor T cells are increasingly used to treat B-cell malignancies.
- Virus-specific T cells are effective in treating and preventing infections in recipients of allogeneic hematopoietic stem cell transplants and in immunosuppressed patients.
- Although many of these cell therapies are manufactured centrally, the cell processing laboratory is involved with shipping, receiving, storing, and infusing these products.

INTRODUCTION

Processing cells and manufacturing cell therapies have been an important part of academic medical centers for more than 30 years. This activity began with the processing of marrow grafts used for hematopoietic progenitor cell (HPC) transplantation. Marrow transplants between ABO-incompatible donor/recipient pairs were problematic because marrow contained large quantities of plasma and red blood cells (RBCs). Initially, transplants involving major donor/recipient ABO incompatibility were performed by using plasma exchange prior to transplantation to lower the recipient's titer of isohemagglutinins and prevent hemolysis. In the 1980s, cell processing laboratories in blood banks began to process marrow to avoid isohemagglutinin-mediated hemolysis related to the transfusion of ABO incompatible RBCs or plasma along with the marrow graft.[1,2] For major ABO incompatibility, hydroxyethyl starch sedimentation in bag systems was used to remove RBCs from the marrow.[1] For minor ABO incompatibility, plasma was removed from the marrow graft by centrifugation and expression, much as plasma is removed from whole blood.

Disclosure Statement: This work was funded by the NIH Clinical Center, Bethesda, Maryland, USA.
Department of Transfusion Medicine, Clinical Center, National Institutes of Health, Center for Cellular Engineering, 10 Center Drive, MSC-1184, Building 10, Room 1C711, Bethesda, MD 20892-1184, USA
* Corresponding author.
E-mail address: dstroncek@cc.nih.gov

Marrow processing laboratories soon began to manufacture novel cell and gene therapies.[2] Early activities included attempts to purge autologous marrow grafts of leukemic cells and the production of autologous gene therapies to treat monogenetic immune deficiencies, such as severe combined immunodeficiency[3] and chronic granulomatous disease.[4] Cell processing laboratories are now manufacturing designer grafts by enriching or depleting certain cell types from bone marrow, umbilical cord blood, and/or mobilized peripheral blood prior to transplantation. For example, enriching grafts for CD34$^+$ cells may facilitate rapid engraftment and lower the incidence of T-cell–mediated graft-versus-host disease (GVHD).[5] Laboratories also are producing marrow-derived and adipose tissue–derived mesenchymal stromal cells for the treatment of acute GVHD and a wide variety of other conditions.[6] Furthermore, they are manufacturing natural killer cell, dendritic cell, and T-cell immunotherapies.

Currently, manufacturing T-cell immunotherapies is one of the major activities of cell processing laboratories. T-cell immunotherapies include donor lymphocyte infusions (DLIs), tumor-infiltrating lymphocytes (TILs), T-cell receptor (TCR)-engineered T cells, chimeric antigen receptor (CAR) T cells, and virus-specific T cells.[7,8] DLIs have been used successfully to manage post-transplant relapses in patients with chronic myeloid leukemia and lymphoma. TIL therapy has been used for many years to treat metastatic melanoma.[9] TCR-engineered T cells are used to treat solid tumors, and CAR T cells to treat B-cell malignancies. Virus-specific T cells are used to treat and prevent Epstein-Barr virus (EBV), cytomegalovirus (CMV), BK virus (BKV), adenovirus, and human herpesvirus 6 (HHV-6) infections in recipients of allogeneic HPC transplants and in other immunosuppressed patients.[10]

This article is focused on T-cell immunotherapies currently used for cancer and virus therapy (**Table 1**). The growth of T-cell immunotherapy has been dramatic over the past 5 years and further growth is expected. The nature and use of these therapies are reviewed. The methods of manufacturing these therapies and the role of the academic center cell processing laboratory that manufactures, stores, and issues these therapies are discussed.

CLINICAL APPLICATION OF T-CELL IMMUNOTHERAPIES
Donor Lymphocyte Infusions

As one of the earliest examples of adoptive immunotherapy, DLIs have been used to treat or prevent relapse of hematologic malignancies after hematopoietic stem cell

Table 1
Types of T-cell immunotherapies, sources of cells used for manufacturing these therapies, and the diseases treated by each specific therapy

Type	Cell Source	Disease
DLIs	Allogeneic PBMNCs	Hematologic malignancies, in particular low-grade leukemia, lymphomas
TILs	Autologous tumors	Metastatic melanoma
TCR-engineered T cells	Autologous peripheral blood lymphocytes	NY-ESO-1–expressing tumors
CAR T cells	Autologous or allogeneic peripheral blood lymphocytes	B-cell malignancies
Virus-specific T cells	Autologous or allogeneic peripheral blood lymphocytes	EBV-associated lymphoproliferative disease, CMV disease, hemorrhagic cystitis, progressive multifocal leukoencephalopathy

transplantation. The therapeutic activity of donor T cells against recipient leukemic cells, or the graft-versus-tumor effect, is enhanced by DLIs in the post-transplant setting. Efficacy was initially reported in chronic myeloid leukemia with up to 70% response rates. Low-grade lymphomas, which relapse post-transplantation, also have been treated successfully with DLIs. Responses are less convincing in high-risk leukemia and myelodysplastic syndromes given the absence of randomized trial data.

DLI also may be used prophylactically to enhance or restore donor chimerism in individuals who do not demonstrate overt relapse post-transplantation. These infusions have been associated, however, with an increased risk of chronic GVHD. More recently, DLIs (with or without concurrent immunosuppression) are under investigation for patients undergoing haploidentical transplantation.[11]

DLIs are manufactured from the mononuclear cell fraction of granulocyte colony-stimulating factor stimulated or unstimulated donor leukapheresis collections. Doses are cryopreserved in aliquots comprising predetermined $CD3^+$ T-cell numbers per kilogram of recipient body weight. They are thawed and administered as needed, as single or multiple infusions after transplantation. Typical doses range from 0.1 to 1×10^6 cells/kg from matched related or unrelated transplant donors.[12]

Tumor-Infiltrating Lymphocytes

TILs are isolated from tumors and expanded over several weeks in culture. TILs have been used for more than 30 years to treat metastatic melanoma[9] and also are being tested in other solid tumors. The overall clinical response rate for melanoma patients treated with TIL ranges from 33% to 56%,[9,13–20] with a complete response of 24% to 29%.[20] Many of these complete responses are of long duration. Up to 20% of all patients have not had relapses after 5 years of therapy.[15,16] Many of the principles of cellular cancer immunotherapy have been developed by clinical investigators who have used TILs to treat melanoma. The clinical response rates of TIL therapy are greater when patients are pretreated with nonmyeloablative leukocyte-reducing chemotherapy.[15] The persistence of TIL cells in the recipients' circulation 1 month after cell infusion is associated with better clinical survival.[16] Finally, TIL expression of the phenotypic marker CD27, a marker of early cellular differentiation, is associated with clinical response.[16]

Additionally, TIL therapy has recently shown some efficacy in treating patients with metastatic human papillomavirus–associated carcinomas. Among 29 patients treated, objective clinical responses have been seen in 5 of 18 (28%) patients with cervical cancer and 2 of 11 (18%) patients with noncervical carcinomas.[21]

Therapy with TILs is not without limitations. TILs cannot be used to treat all patients with melanoma. Some patients do not have tumor that can be resected, and, for some patients, TILs cannot be isolated from the resected tumor. To manufacture TILs, tumor homogenates or fragments are cultured in the presence of interleukin (IL)-2. The autologous T cells are allowed to expand for 14 days to 21 days, and, during expansion, T cells overgrow and kill tumor cells.[22] Some, but not all, of the expanded T cells are reactive to antigens expressed by the tumor. The TILs may be cultured as T-cell clones, and clones that are reactive with tumor cells may undergo further expansion. Alternatively, all T cells may be expanded in bulk. This expansion process, known as the rapid expansion protocol, produces 30 to 60×10^9 TILs over 2 weeks. Rapid expansion protocol involves culturing TIL cells in the presence of feeder cells, IL-2 and anti-CD3. Typically, the feeder cells are peripheral blood mononuclear cells (PBMNCs) from 3 healthy donors that have been pooled and irradiated.[22]

T-cell Receptor–Engineered T Cells

The success of TIL therapy for melanoma has led to clinical trials involving T cells expressing TCRs specific for a variety of tumor antigens. Cancer therapy with TCR-engineered T cells involves collecting PBMNC concentrates by apheresis from an autologous donor, isolating T cells, and then transducing them, followed by expansion of the product. This therapy is limited by the requirement to use TCRs associated with the patients' HLA antigen type. Because TCRs interact with antigen-presenting tumor cells in an HLA-restricted manner, a particular vector can only be used for the treatment of patients with specific HLA antigen types. For example, a tumor-specific TCR isolated from a person with an HLA-A type of HLA-A0201 is effective only in a patient with the HLA type HLA-A0201.

Antigens that have been targeted by TCR-engineered T cells include cancer germline antigens or cancer testis antigens, melanoma antigens, and antigens overexpressed by tumors. Cancer germline antigens are expressed on tumors but not on normal tissue, apart from germline cells, which do not express HLA antigens.[13] Adoptive cellular therapy using T cells engineered to express TCRs reactive with cancer antigens has shown variable efficacy and toxicity profiles, depending on the target antigen.

Cancer testis antigens include MAGE-A3 and NY-ESO-1. Immunotherapy with T cells engineered to express TCRs reactive with MAGE-A3 has been associated with some clinical efficacy, although along with significant off-target toxicity.[23] T cells engineered to express TCRs specific to NY-ESO-1 have been effective and less toxic. NY-ESO-1 is expressed on 70% to 80% of synovial cell sarcoma and 10% to 50% of melanoma, lung, breast, prostate, thyroid, and ovarian cancers.[24] T cells engineered to express a TCR specific for NY-ESO-1 have been used to treat patients with melanoma and synovial cell sarcoma. Among 20 patients with NY-ESO-1+ melanoma in this trial, 11 (55%) had objective clinical responses and an estimated 5-year overall survival of 33%. For 18 patients with NY-ESO-1+ synovial cell sarcoma, 61% had objective clinical responses and the estimated 5-year overall survival rate was 14%.[24]

Treatment of cancer with engineered T cells expressing TCRs specific for melanoma differentiation antigens and antigens overexpressed in tumors also has been associated with significant toxicity. T cells directed at the melanoma differentiation antigens gp100 and MART-1 have been tested in clinical trials in patients with melanoma.[25] Because melanoma differentiation antigens are expressed on both melanoma tumor cells and normal melanocytic cells, targeting these antigens in this study was associated with the destruction of normal tissues where melanocytes are found, including the skin, eyes, and inner ears.

Chimeric Antigen Receptor T Cells

CAR T cells are engineered to express a construct that includes a single chain variable fragment (scFv) of an antibody directed to a tumor-specific antigen, the signaling portion of the TCR, the CD3 zeta chain, a hinge region, and a CD8 binding domain. In addition, a T-cell costimulatory molecule is included, such as CD28 or 4-1BB (CD137).[26] To manufacture CAR T cells, autologous PBMNCs are collected by apheresis, T cells are isolated from the apheresis concentrate, and T cells then are transduced and expanded over 7 days to 10 days.

CAR T cells are self-contained in that the binding of the antibody portion of the transgene activates T cells without the need for engagement of a costimulatory or HLA class I molecule. Because antibodies are not HLA restricted, 1 CAR construct can be used to treat all individuals regardless of their HLA antigen type. Additionally, because CAR T cells bind to their target via scFv, the target antigen does not have to be processed by HLA molecules and loss of expression of HLA molecules by tumors does not prevent CAR T cell–mediated cytotoxicity.

CAR T cells are clinically effective for the treatment of B-cell leukemia and lymphomas. CD19-CAR T cells are used to treat B-cell lymphoma,[27–32] B-cell acute lymphoblastic leukemia (ALL),[33] and chronic lymphocytic leukemia.[34,35] The overall response rates have been 64% to 83% for patients with refractory B cell lymphomas,[30,31,36] with a complete response rate of 43% to 71%.[30,31,36] The overall remission rate for children and young adults with ALL treated with CD19-CAR T cells was 81% and the complete response rate was 60%.[32] For chronic lymphocytic leukemia, 1 study of 14 patients reported an overall response rate of 57%, with complete responses seen in 4 patients.[35]

Several other CAR T cells directed against B cells are in clinical trials. CD22-CAR T cells are effective in treating children and young adults with ALL whose cells do not express CD19,[37] and anti–B-cell maturation antigen (BCMA) CAR T cells are used to treat patients with multiple myeloma.[38,39] Among 15 patients with ALL treated with greater than or equal to 1×10^6 CD22-CAR T cells per kilogram, 11 (73%) had a complete response with a median relapse-free survival of 6 months.[37] The clinical response rate of 16 patients with multiple myeloma treated with 9×10^6 anti-BCMA CAR T cells per kilogram was 81%, with a very good partial response or complete response in 63%.[39]

CAR T cells are living cells. After infusion, CAR T cells expand in vivo and reach peak levels after 1 week to 2 weeks. During the period of in vivo CAR T-cell expansion, the recipient can develop cytokine release syndrome (CRS).[40,41] CRS is associated with fever, hypotension, capillary leak syndrome, organ failure, coagulopathy, and hemophagocytic lymphohistiocytosis. Cell expansion is associated with target cell lysis and elevation of a wide variety of factors.[39] The levels of many factors, including IL-6, IL-8, IL-10, IL-15, and interferon-γ, are correlated with severity of CRS.[33,39] The development of CRS has been associated with clinical response to CAR T-cell therapy. Patients with greater tumor burden and greater CAR T-cell expansion in vivo are more likely to experience severe CRS. Tocilizumab, an anti–IL-6 receptor antibody, is used to treat severe CRS. If tocilizumab therapy is not effective, steroids can be used.

Recipients of CAR T-cell therapy also can experience neurotoxicity or CAR T-cell–related encephalopathy syndrome (CRES).[40,42] CRES is associated with headache, confusion, and speech disturbance. It can progress to seizures, focal defects, and cerebral edema. Its pathophysiology is less certain, but it is associated with a combination of factors, including the activation of central nervous system endothelial cells with the subsequent breakdown of the blood-brain barrier, elevated cytokine levels in the central nervous system, and cerebral infiltration by T cells.[42]

Virus-Specific T Cells

Virus-specific T cells were first used to treat and prevent infections in patients who were immunosuppressed after HPC transplantation. Initially, these cells were used treat EBV-associated lymphoproliferative disease after allogeneic HPC transplantation.[43,44] Later, they were used to treat CMV infections in transplant recipients. Virus-specific T cells are now used to treat and prevent several viral infections, including EBV, CMV, adenovirus, BKV, and HHV-6. Recently, they have been used to treat viral infections in immunosuppressed patients. Preliminary clinical trials suggest that virus-specific T cells may be effective in treating progressive multifocal leukoencephalopathy due to the polyomavirus, JC virus.[10]

Virus-specific T cells have been manufactured using several different methods. All methods use PBMNCs as a source of T cells. A wide variety of sources of viral antigens have been used to sensitize T cells. EBV-transformed T cells have been used to sensitize T cells to EBV. EBV-transformed T cells have been transduced with adenovirus vectors encoding immune dominant proteins of other viruses, such as CMV pp65 or CMV immediate early 1 (IE-1), which allows these cells to sensitize other T cells to CMV or other viruses.[45] These EBV-transformed adenovirus vector-transduced cells also prime T cells to EBV and adenovirus. More recently, pools of overlapping peptides derived from immune dominant viral proteins have been used for T-cell sensitization.[46,47]

Some virus-specific T-cell manufacturing methods make use of dendritic cells prepared from the PBMNCs.[48] The dendritic cells are used to process and present viral peptides. Alternatively, T cells can be sensitized to peptides using irradiated autologous PBMNCs as antigen-presenting cells.[46,47]

It also is possible to isolate virus-specific T cells directly from donor PBMNCs using immune dominant viral peptides associated with HLA tetramers that bind to the TCR of the virus-specific T cells. Another method involves stimulating PBMNCs with viral peptides and capturing sensitized T cells using antibodies directed to activation markers or cytokines. Both of these methods, however, are costly.

Originally, manufacturing virus-specific T cells was a lengthy process that required many weeks.[10] The manufacturing process has changed, and, currently, these cells can be produced in approximately 2 weeks using autologous antigen-presenting cells and viral peptide libraries.[10,46,47]

Classically, virus-specific T cells were produced from PBMNCs collected from the HPC transplant donor or, for patients with progressive multifocal leukoencephalopathy, from an HLA-compatible relative. Because viral infections in immunosuppressed patients require prompt treatment, recently, banks of virus-specific T cells have been produced from HLA-typed healthy subjects.[49,50] These third-party virus-specific T cells are cryopreserved and stored and are available for use as an off-the-shelf therapy. Partially HLA-matched virus-specific cells are used to treat patients when the clinical need arises.

Off-the-shelf virus-specific T cells have been used to treat BKV, HHV-6, CMV, EBV, and adenovirus infections after allogeneic HPC transplantation. Among 38 patients treated with off-the-shelf virus-specific T cells, 92% had a complete or partial clinical response.[50] The clinical response rate for specific viruses was 100% for BKV (n = 16), 94% for CMV (n = 17), 71% for adenovirus (n = 7), and 100% for EBV (n = 2).[50] Thirteen of the 14 patients treated for BKV-associated hemorrhagic cystitis experienced resolution of gross hematuria. The third-party donor virus-specific T cells were observed in the circulation of the recipients for up to 12 weeks. Two patients experienced mild de novo skin GVHD (grade 1), 1 patient developed recurrent upper gastrointestinal GVHD, and 3 patients developed recurrent grade 1 or grade 2 skin GVHD. None of the recipients developed CRS.[50]

OVERVIEW OF SPECIFIC METHODS USED FOR THE PRODUCTION OF T-CELL IMMUNOTHERAPIES

The methods used to produce T-cell immunotherapies are dependent on the clinical use of the therapy, but there are many commonalities (**Table 2**). First, PBMNCs are collected through the process of leukapheresis. They are then enriched for T cells, which can be stimulated using a variety of techniques and expanded in culture for several days. In most cases, the T cells are transduced with viral vectors encoding

Table 2
Steps, processes, and materials involved in manufacturing T-cell immunotherapies

Step	Processes/Materials
Cell collection	Phlebotomy Apheresis
T-cell enrichment	Density gradient separation Counter-flow elutriation Antibody selection
Cell expansion—vessel	Bags Bioreactors
Cell expansion—stimulation	IL-2 plus anti-CD3 IL-2 plus anti-CD3/anti-CD28 beads
Cell washing and concentration	Centrifuge Automated cell washers

CAR or TCR constructs; however, some manufacturing centers are pursuing nonviral integration through transposase systems. At the end of the culture period, the cells are washed and concentrated and then undergo lot release testing. The final T-cell product may be infused fresh or it may be cryopreserved and infused after several days or months of storage. The operations involved with the production of T-cell immunotherapies are reviewed later.

Closed System Processing

Cell and gene therapies, including T-cell immunotherapies, are manufactured in highly controlled facilities specifically designed for this purpose, where aseptic processing techniques are used to reduce the risk of microbial contamination of the cells. To further ensure the sterility of the cellular therapies, closed systems, which were pioneered in blood banking, are used whenever possible.

Future closed system manufacturing will likely use automated bioreactors. These advanced instruments are capable of washing, selecting, transducing, expanding, and harvesting T cells in 1 easy-to-use benchtop device. The authors and other investigators have already begun to incorporate these instruments into manufacturing facilities and currently are implementing them for clinical manufacturing for ongoing trials.[51–53] These types of instruments are attractive not only because they are closed system devices that improve sterile culture but also because they have the potential to optimize manufacturing space in costly clean rooms and minimize labor time as well as costs.

Collection of Leukocytes

Although many people may have an adequate quantity of lymphocytes for manufacturing T-cell immunotherapies in as little as a few hundred milliliters of blood, the quantity of circulating lymphocytes is highly variable. Consequently, PBMNCs typically are collected by apheresis using blood cell separators that have been specifically designed to collect leukocytes. Blood cell separators draw venous whole blood, separate mononuclear leukocytes from other blood cells based on cell density, and return RBCs, platelets, and plasma back to the donor through a separate vein.

Because the size and density of T cells are similar to those of other leukocytes, the leukocytes collected by apheresis not only are rich in T cells but also can contain considerable quantities of B cells, monocytes, and natural killer cells. PBMNC concentrates also contain some platelets, RBCs, and granulocytes. The degree of platelet and RBC contamination generally is consistent, but the granulocyte content is more variable, with some apheresis concentrates containing few, if any, granulocytes, and others containing larger quantities. Because it is important to begin manufacturing with a leukocyte population that has a high proportion of T cells, the PBMNCs must undergo T-cell enrichment.

T-cell Enrichment

PBMNC concentrates are enriched for lymphocytes to eliminate cells that may inhibit T-cell expansion or compete for vector. Several methods are being used for T-cell enrichment, including density gradient separation, counter-flow elutriation, and monoclonal antibody selection. The effectiveness and techniques of these 3 methods vary considerably.

Automated instruments are available for closed system density gradient separation, counter-flow elutriation, and monoclonal antibody separation.[54–56] These instruments utilize 1-time use, closed system sterile disposable sets. Cells come in contact only with the disposable sets, and a new set is used for each procedure to minimize the risk of cross-contaminating cells or infectious agents from 1 patient to another. Because of the disposable nature of the kits, these instruments can be prepared quickly for processing cells from a new patient.

T-cell Transduction

The production of many T-cell immunotherapies involves T-cell transduction with gamma-retroviral or lentiviral vectors. The cells are transduced once or twice and result in expression of the vector in 20% to 80% or more of the T cells. T cells also can be manufactured with nonintegrated plasmids or messenger RNA. CAR T cells transduced with transiently expressed vectors may need to be given on multiple occasions. Closed system methods are available for the gamma-retroviral and lentiviral vector transduction of T cells.[57] Gamma-retroviral transduction requires T-cell division, and, as such, T cells are stimulated or activated for 2 days or 3 days prior to transduction. Lentiviral vector transduction does not require cell division, but T cells typically are stimulated for a day prior to lentiviral transduction.

T-cell Expansion

T cells often are expanded by stimulation with anti-CD3 antibodies and the cytokine IL-2. Anti-CD3 and anti-CD28 may be attached to magnetic beads, which stimulate the TCR and the CD28 costimulatory molecule to allow the beads to act as artificial antigen-presenting cells.[58] These anti-CD3/anti-CD28 beads and IL-2 commonly are used to stimulated T-cell expansion. At the end of cell expansion, the magnetic beads may need to be removed from the CAR T cells.

Classically, T cells were cultured in flasks. Bags and other closed systems have replaced flasks for T-cell culture and expansion. Bag systems are easy to use and can be adopted for many clinical cell processing applications. They are limited, however, by the fact that cells are cultured at a relatively low density of 1 to 2×10^6 cells/mL.

Flasks with gas permeable membranes have also been designed for culturing T cells at densities up to 5 to 6×10^6 cells/mL.[22] These flasks are available with integral tubes that can be used for closed system processing.

POST-MANUFACTURING OR DOWNSTREAM PROCESSING

The cell processing laboratory is involved with several steps after the completion of manufacturing. The cells are washed and suspended in an infusible solution. Samples then are taken for lot release testing. In some cases, the harvested cells are infused within a few hours, but, in most cases, the final cellular therapy is cryopreserved and stored until the results of lot release testing are available. These steps are similar for all types of T-cell immunotherapies.

T-cell Harvest

Once T-cell expansion is complete, the cells are washed to remove cytokines, media, and media supplements that may be toxic to the patient when administered intravenously. The cells are then resuspended in a solution that can be given intravenously, such as Plasma-Lyte A with albumin.

Laboratory Testing of the Final T-cell Product

For autologous therapies, the cells manufactured for each patient are considered a new lot of cells and they are tested at the end of manufacturing. This testing is known as lot release testing. Lot release testing includes identity, safety, and potency testing. The cells are tested for sterility using bacterial and fungal culture assays. If the cells are to be given immediately after they are washed and concentrated, they are tested for endotoxin and are evaluated by Gram stain.

Cryopreservation

Although some T-cell immunotherapies are infused immediately after they are harvested, most are cryopreserved and stored, then thawed when ready to be infused. When cryopreservation is needed, cells are aliquoted into the appropriate dose, a cryoprotectant is added, and the cells are cryopreserved. The purpose of the cryoprotectant is to prevent damage to the cells by ice crystal formation during the freeze-thaw process. To further improve the recovery of cells at the time of thaw and infusion, the cells typically are cryopreserved using a programmable freezer that controls the rate of temperature change. After cryopreservation, the cells generally are stored in liquid nitrogen or the vapor phase of liquid nitrogen.

CELL THERAPY INFUSION

Much as with blood transfusion, when cellular therapies are to be administered to the patient, the clinical care team orders the cells, and the processing laboratory issues the cells to the patient care unit. When T-cell therapies have been cryopreserved, they must be thawed before they are issued. The cells are thawed rapidly, and, once thawed, the cells must be infused as soon as possible as the dimethyl sulfoxide used in most cryoprotectants is toxic to the cells.

The time in which the infusion begins and ends is documented by nursing staff. The patient's vital signs also are documented before, during, and after the infusion. The recipient also should be monitored for reactions associated with cell infusions. Cell therapy reactions can manifest as fever, chills, or a change in pulse, blood pressure, or respiratory rate. Reactions to the cellular therapy product typically occur within hours of administration. Reactions may be to the cells, cellular debris, or dimethyl sulfoxide.

Reactions associated with T-cell expansion, such as CRS and CRES, occur within 1 day to 14 days post-infusion. These reactions are not a direct result of the infusion of the T cells; rather, they are a consequence of T-cell expansion and cytotoxicity. Both immediate and intermediate toxicities may be managed by joint consultation with the immunotherapy, transplantation, and transfusion medicine teams.

SUMMARY

T-cell immunotherapies are an important part of clinical medicine, and cell therapy laboratories have become an integral part of the modern health care center. Cell therapy laboratories are involved with receiving starting material and with processing and culturing cells to create the immunotherapy product. They also test, store, thaw, and issue the final product. In addition, the cell therapy laboratory has an important role in the evaluation of reactions associated with the infusion of these cellular therapies.

REFERENCES

1. Warkentin PI, Hilden JM, Kersey JH, et al. Transplantation of major ABO-incompatible bone marrow depleted of red cells by hydroxyethyl starch. Vox Sang 1985;48(2):89–104.
2. McCullough J. Collection and use of stem cells; role of transfusion centers in bone marrow transplantation. Vox Sang 1994;67(Suppl 3):35–42.
3. Blaese RM, Culver KW, Miller AD, et al. T lymphocyte-directed gene therapy for ADA- SCID: initial trial results after 4 years. Science 1995;270(5235):475–80.
4. Malech HL, Maples PB, Whiting-Theobald N, et al. Prolonged production of NADPH oxidase-corrected granulocytes after gene therapy of chronic granulomatous disease. Proc Natl Acad Sci U S A 1997;94(22):12133–8.
5. Avecilla ST, Goss C, Bleau S, et al. How do I perform hematopoietic progenitor cell selection? Transfusion 2016;56(5):1008–12.
6. Fisher SA, Cutler A, Doree C, et al. Mesenchymal stromal cells as treatment or prophylaxis for acute or chronic graft-versus-host disease in haematopoietic stem cell transplant (HSCT) recipients with a haematological condition. Cochrane Database Syst Rev 2019;(1):CD009768.
7. Met O, Jensen KM, Chamberlain CA, et al. Principles of adoptive T cell therapy in cancer. Semin Immunopathol 2019;41(1):49–58.
8. Ikeda H. T-cell adoptive immunotherapy using tumor-infiltrating T cells and genetically engineered TCR-T cells. Int Immunol 2016;28(7):349–53.
9. Rosenberg SA, Packard BS, Aebersold PM, et al. Use of tumor-infiltrating lymphocytes and interleukin-2 in the immunotherapy of patients with metastatic melanoma. A preliminary report. N Engl J Med 1988;319(25):1676–80.
10. Barrett AJ, Prockop S, Bollard CM. Reprint of: virus-specific T cells: broadening applicability. Biol Blood Marrow Transplant 2018;24(3S):S1–6.
11. Toprak SK. Donor lymphocyte infusion in myeloid disorders. Transfus Apher Sci 2018;57(2):178–86.
12. Zeiser R, Beelen DW, Bethge W, et al. Biology-driven approaches to prevent and treat relapse of myeloid neoplasia after allogeneic hematopoietic stem cell transplantation. Biol Blood Marrow Transplant 2019;25(4):e128–40.
13. Rosenberg SA, Restifo NP. Adoptive cell transfer as personalized immunotherapy for human cancer. Science 2015;348(6230):62–8.
14. Rosenberg SA, Yannelli JR, Yang JC, et al. Treatment of patients with metastatic melanoma with autologous tumor-infiltrating lymphocytes and interleukin 2. J Natl Cancer Inst 1994;86(15):1159–66.
15. Dudley ME, Wunderlich JR, Robbins PF, et al. Cancer regression and autoimmunity in patients after clonal repopulation with antitumor lymphocytes. Science 2002;298(5594):850–4.
16. Rosenberg SA, Yang JC, Sherry RM, et al. Durable complete responses in heavily pretreated patients with metastatic melanoma using T-cell transfer immunotherapy. Clin Cancer Res 2011;17(13):4550–7.

17. Radvanyi LG, Bernatchez C, Zhang M, et al. Specific lymphocyte subsets predict response to adoptive cell therapy using expanded autologous tumor-infiltrating lymphocytes in metastatic melanoma patients. Clin Cancer Res 2012;18(24): 6758–70.
18. Pilon-Thomas S, Kuhn L, Ellwanger S, et al. Efficacy of adoptive cell transfer of tumor-infiltrating lymphocytes after lymphopenia induction for metastatic melanoma. J Immunother 2012;35(8):615–20.
19. Besser MJ, Shapira-Frommer R, Itzhaki O, et al. Adoptive transfer of tumor-infiltrating lymphocytes in patients with metastatic melanoma: intent-to-treat analysis and efficacy after failure to prior immunotherapies. Clin Cancer Res 2013; 19(17):4792–800.
20. Goff SL, Dudley ME, Citrin DE, et al. Randomized, prospective evaluation comparing intensity of lymphodepletion before adoptive transfer of tumor-infiltrating lymphocytes for patients with metastatic melanoma. J Clin Oncol 2016;34(20):2389–97.
21. Stevanovic S, Helman SR, Wunderlich JR, et al. A phase II study of tumor-infiltrating lymphocyte therapy for human papillomavirus-associated epithelial cancers. Clin Cancer Res 2019;25(5):1486–93.
22. Jin J, Sabatino M, Somerville R, et al. Simplified method of the growth of human tumor infiltrating lymphocytes in gas-permeable flasks to numbers needed for patient treatment. J Immunother 2012;35(3):283–92.
23. Morgan RA, Chinnasamy N, Abate-Daga D, et al. Cancer regression and neurological toxicity following anti-MAGE-A3 TCR gene therapy. J Immunother 2013; 36(2):133–51.
24. Robbins PF, Kassim SH, Tran TL, et al. A pilot trial using lymphocytes genetically engineered with an NY-ESO-1-reactive T-cell receptor: long-term follow-up and correlates with response. Clin Cancer Res 2015;21(5):1019–27.
25. Johnson LA, Morgan RA, Dudley ME, et al. Gene therapy with human and mouse T-cell receptors mediates cancer regression and targets normal tissues expressing cognate antigen. Blood 2009;114(3):535–46.
26. Boyiadzis MM, Dhodapkar MV, Brentjens RJ, et al. Chimeric antigen receptor (CAR) T therapies for the treatment of hematologic malignancies: clinical perspective and significance. J Immunother Cancer 2018;6(1):137.
27. Kochenderfer JN, Wilson WH, Janik JE, et al. Eradication of B-lineage cells and regression of lymphoma in a patient treated with autologous T cells genetically engineered to recognize CD19. Blood 2010;116(20):4099–102.
28. Kochenderfer JN, Dudley ME, Kassim SH, et al. Chemotherapy-refractory diffuse large B-cell lymphoma and indolent B-cell malignancies can be effectively treated with autologous T cells expressing an anti-CD19 chimeric antigen receptor. J Clin Oncol 2015;33(6):540–9.
29. Brudno JN, Somerville RP, Shi V, et al. Allogeneic T cells that express an anti-CD19 chimeric antigen receptor induce remissions of B-cell malignancies that progress after allogeneic hematopoietic stem-cell transplantation without causing graft-versus-host disease. J Clin Oncol 2016;34(10):1112–21.
30. Neelapu SS, Locke FL, Bartlett NL, et al. Axicabtagene ciloleucel car T-cell therapy in refractory large B-cell lymphoma. N Engl J Med 2017;377(26):2531–44.
31. Locke FL, Ghobadi A, Jacobson CA, et al. Long-term safety and activity of axicabtagene ciloleucel in refractory large B-cell lymphoma (ZUMA-1): a single-arm, multicentre, phase 1-2 trial. Lancet Oncol 2019;20(1):31–42.
32. Maude SL, Laetsch TW, Buechner J, et al. Tisagenlecleucel in children and young adults with B-cell lymphoblastic leukemia. N Engl J Med 2018;378(5):439–48.

33. Lee DW, Kochenderfer JN, Stetler-Stevenson M, et al. T cells expressing CD19 chimeric antigen receptors for acute lymphoblastic leukaemia in children and young adults: a phase 1 dose-escalation trial. Lancet 2015;385(9967):517–28.

34. Kochenderfer JN, Dudley ME, Carpenter RO, et al. Donor-derived CD19-targeted T cells cause regression of malignancy persisting after allogeneic hematopoietic stem cell transplantation. Blood 2013;122(25):4129–39.

35. Porter DL, Hwang WT, Frey NV, et al. Chimeric antigen receptor T cells persist and induce sustained remissions in relapsed refractory chronic lymphocytic leukemia. Sci Transl Med 2015;7(303):303ra139.

36. Schuster SJ, Svoboda J, Chong EA, et al. Chimeric antigen receptor T cells in refractory B-cell lymphomas. N Engl J Med 2017;377(26):2545–54.

37. Fry TJ, Shah NN, Orentas RJ, et al. CD22-targeted CAR T cells induce remission in B-ALL that is naive or resistant to CD19-targeted CAR immunotherapy. Nat Med 2018;24(1):20–8.

38. Ali SA, Shi V, Maric I, et al. T cells expressing an anti-B-cell maturation antigen chimeric antigen receptor cause remissions of multiple myeloma. Blood 2016; 128(13):1688–700.

39. Brudno JN, Maric I, Hartman SD, et al. T cells genetically modified to express an anti-B-cell maturation antigen chimeric antigen receptor cause remissions of poor-prognosis relapsed multiple myeloma. J Clin Oncol 2018;36(22):2267–80.

40. Brudno JN, Kochenderfer JN. Recent advances in CAR T-cell toxicity: mechanisms, manifestations and management. Blood Rev 2019;34:45–55.

41. Brudno JN, Kochenderfer JN. Toxicities of chimeric antigen receptor T cells: recognition and management. Blood 2016;127(26):3321–30.

42. Mahadeo KM, Khazal SJ, Abdel-Azim H, et al. Management guidelines for paediatric patients receiving chimeric antigen receptor T cell therapy. Nat Rev Clin Oncol 2019;16(1):45–63.

43. Heslop HE, Rooney CM. Adoptive cellular immunotherapy for EBV lymphoproliferative disease. Immunol Rev 1997;157:217–22.

44. Heslop HE, Slobod KS, Pule MA, et al. Long-term outcome of EBV-specific T-cell infusions to prevent or treat EBV-related lymphoproliferative disease in transplant recipients. Blood 2010;115(5):925–35.

45. Hanley PJ, Shaffer DR, Cruz CR, et al. Expansion of T cells targeting multiple antigens of cytomegalovirus, Epstein-Barr virus and adenovirus to provide broad antiviral specificity after stem cell transplantation. Cytotherapy 2011;13(8): 976–86.

46. Gerdemann U, Keirnan JM, Katari UL, et al. Rapidly generated multivirus-specific cytotoxic T lymphocytes for the prophylaxis and treatment of viral infections. Mol Ther 2012;20(8):1622–32.

47. Nishiyama-Fujita Y, Kawana-Tachikawa AI, Ono T, et al. Generation of multivirus-specific T cells by a single stimulation of peripheral blood mononuclear cells with a peptide mixture using serum-free medium. Cytotherapy 2018;20(9):1182–90.

48. Hanley PJ, Cruz CR, Savoldo B, et al. Functionally active virus-specific T cells that target CMV, adenovirus, and EBV can be expanded from naive T-cell populations in cord blood and will target a range of viral epitopes. Blood 2009;114(9): 1958–67.

49. Leen AM, Bollard CM, Mendizabal AM, et al. Multicenter study of banked third-party virus-specific T cells to treat severe viral infections after hematopoietic stem cell transplantation. Blood 2013;121(26):5113–23.

50. Tzannou I, Papadopoulou A, Naik S, et al. Off-the-shelf virus-specific T cells to treat BK virus, human herpesvirus 6, cytomegalovirus, epstein-barr virus, and

adenovirus infections after allogeneic hematopoietic stem-cell transplantation. J Clin Oncol 2017;35(31):3547–57.

51. Mock U, Nickolay L, Philip B, et al. Automated manufacturing of chimeric antigen receptor T cells for adoptive immunotherapy using CliniMACS prodigy. Cytotherapy 2016;18(8):1002–11.

52. Lock D, Mockel-Tenbrinck N, Drechsel K, et al. Automated manufacturing of potent CD20-directed chimeric antigen receptor T cells for clinical use. Hum Gene Ther 2017;28(10):914–25.

53. Zhu F, Shah N, Xu H, et al. Closed-system manufacturing of CD19 and dual-targeted CD20/19 chimeric antigen receptor T cells using the CliniMACS Prodigy device at an academic medical center. Cytotherapy 2018;20(3):394–406.

54. Stroncek DF, Lee DW, Ren J, et al. Elutriated lymphocytes for manufacturing chimeric antigen receptor T cells. J Transl Med 2017;15(1):59.

55. Sabatino M, Hu J, Sommariva M, et al. Generation of clinical-grade CD19-specific CAR-modified CD8+ memory stem cells for the treatment of human B-cell malignancies. Blood 2016;128(4):519–28.

56. Turtle CJ, Hanafi LA, Berger C, et al. CD19 CAR-T cells of defined CD4+:CD8+ composition in adult B cell ALL patients. J Clin Invest 2016;126(6):2123–38.

57. Jin J, Gkitsas N, Fellowes VS, et al. Enhanced clinical-scale manufacturing of TCR transduced T-cells using closed culture system modules. J Transl Med 2018;16(1):13.

58. Tumaini B, Lee DW, Lin T, et al. Simplified process for the production of anti-CD19-CAR-engineered T cells. Cytotherapy 2013;15(11):1406–15.

Current and Future Cell Therapy Standards and Guidelines

J. Wade Atkins, MS, MT(ASCP) SBB, CQA(ASQ)[a],*, Kamille West, MD[b],
Kimberly A. Kasow, DO[c]

KEYWORDS

- Cellular therapies • Biologic drug products • HCT/Ps • Licensure requirements
- PHS 351 and 361

KEY POINTS

- Cell biologists and cellular engineers are creating powerful cell-based biologic drugs that hold promise for treating serious conditions and genetic defects.
- Biologic products may pose higher risk of transmission of communicable disease from contamination or cross contamination or donor sources.
- Engineered cellular products may pose higher risk of serious adverse events from expansion or modifications.
- Regulations and practice standards are evolving to address safety concerns as these biologic drug products are being quickly introduced into the market.

INTRODUCTION

The practice of using cellular products collected from a patient or an allogenic donor to treat a disease or modify defects within a patient's genome is rapidly expanding in biotherapeutic medicine. The first successful bone marrow transplant (BMT) between an identical twin pair in 1956 by Dr E. Donnall Thomas to treat leukemia[1] followed by a successful BMT to treat an infant with an immune deficiency syndrome using a human leukocyte antigen–matched sibling donor[2] in 1968 performed by Giatti and Good initiated the development of cellular-based therapeutic drugs. Using these products as drugs to treat leukemias and other gene-based diseases has opened up new therapy

Disclosure: No financial disclosures reported by any of the authors.
[a] Department of Transfusion Medicine, Clinical Center, NIH, 10 Center Drive, MSC-1184, Building 10, Room 1C/711B, Bethesda, MD 20892-1184, USA; [b] Blood Services, Department of Transfusion Medicine, Clinical Center, NIH, 10 Center Drive, MSC-1184, Building 10, Room 1C/711E, Bethesda, MD 20892-1184, USA; [c] Department of Pediatrics, University of North Carolina, 1108 Physicians Office Building, 170 Manning, Drive, CB 7236, Chapel Hill, NC 27599-7236, USA
* Corresponding author.
E-mail address: jatkins@cc.nih.gov

Hematol Oncol Clin N Am 33 (2019) 839–855
https://doi.org/10.1016/j.hoc.2019.05.008
0889-8588/19/Published by Elsevier Inc.

hemonc.theclinics.com

approaches beyond chemotherapy and surgery. These emerging cellular therapies use hematopoietic stem cells (HSCs), less differentiated cell lines, and more mature cells. Immature, pluripotent stem cells, stromal cells, mesenchymal cells, and T lymphocytes are some of the cell lines being used as source material for manufacturing biologic drug products. Targeted cell populations can be expanded by culture methods or modified by gene manipulations or insertions and are being studied to determine whether these products are safe for human use in a variety of diseases. Although these products are intended to treat disease, cellular therapies have risks. With this upsurge in research and clinical advancements, the US Food and Drug Administration (FDA) must balance its duties between advancing treatment and heath care options and ensuring the safety and quality of drugs, including biologic products, being introduced for patient use.

CURRENT CELLULAR THERAPIES AND APPROACHES

Research into cell lines, their function, and possible usage as therapeutic drugs is quickly evolving. Many sources exist for stem cells, such as the bone marrow, brain, blood, skeletal and cardiac muscle, skin, and liver. Although HSC transplant is the most commonly used cell therapy, other cell types, such as mesenchymal stem cells (MSCs), are being used to treat various diseases. Cell populations may be expanded in culture, genetically altered, modified, or a combination of manufacturing processes to harness the power of immunotherapy. The use of embryonic stem cells (ESCs) is still controversial because of ethical and political concerns surrounding their source. ESCs may yield more applications in the future because of their pluripotent state, which may allow scientists and cellular engineers more options to develop therapeutic products. These cellular manipulations, modifications, and less differentiated cell lines hold great promise but inherently pose greater risks.

As cell biologists develop a greater understanding of cellular and genetic properties and functions of these cell groups, they are able to quickly share this information in the digital age. Cellular engineering scientists have faster access to this published information and can quickly develop potential therapeutic applications. The increasing rate and shortened interval between published, peer-reviewed studies is driving innovation at a fast pace. This progress is creating a need for carefully developed regulations, guidance documents, educational seminars, and consensus standards for clinical practices for maximum patient safety. The onslaught of scientific discoveries and distribution of new and additional regulatory guidance and accreditation standards can be overwhelming. Balance is needed to safely move the development of cellular therapy drug products and their clinical use forward because critically ill patients are in need of these innovative approaches.

HSCs were originally harvested from the bone marrow for transplant and these products continue to be regulated under the Health Resources and Services Administration solid organ transplant rules, which at that time were the only regulations for safely transplanting human cells or organs. These regulations adequately provide for safe and effective medical practice when no manipulation to the marrow product occurs. Solid organs and unmanipulated bone marrow are not subject to biologics licensure regulations or interstate commerce rules.

In contrast, cord blood products provide the same therapeutic effect as bone marrow–derived products but are subject to licensure laws. Cord and all other cellular products are regulated through different pathways than unmanipulated bone marrow products because of the risks associated with the preparation, manipulation, or modification steps. The risk association and increasing potential for harm from contamination, cross contamination, mix-up, and spread of communicable disease is the basis for current regulatory pathways.

MANIPULATIONS AND MODIFICATIONS

Bone marrow, cord blood, and peripheral blood stem cells have been extensively studied and used to reconstitute hematopoietic cellular function for decades. This experience allows:

- Greater understanding of therapeutic function of well-characterized products
- Identification of the risks in allogeneic use and development of effective risk mitigation strategies to prevent known complications such as graft-versus-host disease or graft rejection
- Confidence that these unmanipulated products can be safely used with less stringent regulatory oversight

MSCs are another promising avenue for emerging cellular therapy products, and understanding the characteristics and function of these cells has simultaneously raised hopes and concerns in cellular tissue engineering. MSCs can be differentiated into bone, cartilage, fat, neurons, pancreas, cardiac and lung cells, astrocytes, and endothelial cells under appropriate ex vivo stimulatory conditions. MSC plasticity is intriguing to cellular engineers and is being evaluated for regenerative medicine approaches such as cellular repair of cardiac muscle after an infarction. Induced pluripotent stem cells (iPSCs), derived from differentiated somatic cells, can also be reprogrammed using electroporation (pulsing) or stimulant cultures, causing them to revert to a less differentiated pluripotent state. These cells can then be coaxed into developing into different therapeutic cell lines. For example, cells expressing CD34 can be pulsed back to an immature state and reprogrammed by culture with cytokines to become pigmented retinal cells.[3]

The ability to reprogram MSCs and iPSCS has profoundly affected research strategies for treatment options. Bench research has provided insight into cell fate mechanisms, identification of key influencing cytokines, gene expression regulators, and control mechanisms driving cell differentiation in controlled conditions, which raises hope that manipulation of cells may offer more sustained therapeutic options. Ex vivo cell manipulation is less well understood than unmanipulated graft products. This lack of information leads to increased uncertainty and risk when these products are used in humans and requires carefully vetted, peer-reviewed clinical trials with safety monitors.

More recently, gene therapy (GT) researchers have made important breakthroughs by either inserting modified, corrected genes into the genome or manipulating the patient's genome. GT ex vivo techniques are used to transfer genetic material into cells through a vector to modify transcriptional expression and correct pathologic defects. Recent ex vivo GT trials have only been conducted using inactivated viral vectors with impaired replication. This viral nonreplicating gene transfer vector is a safety strategy to prevent unintended viral disease and oncogenesis.

Gene editing procedures alter DNA sequences using artificially modified nucleases, which act as a molecular scissor and can be used as a DNA repair mechanism or induce insertions and deletions of gene sequences. Recent advances in genome editing have been made using CRISPR (clustered regularly interspaced short palindromic repeats)-Cas9 technology as a method to repair gene sequences.[4]

An example of gene modification is T lymphocytes that have been engineered to act as cancer cell killers. These chimeric antigen receptor (CAR) T cells are modified immune cells with an engineered receptor to an antigen or target site on the cancer cell.

REGULATORY STRUCTURE: HISTORIC AND CURRENT UNITED STATES REGULATIONS

As researchers continue to understand cellular maturation and function and cellular engineers are creating more investigational products, the safety, quality, identity, purity, and potency of these novel products are of essential importance. Regulatory pathways provide for both public health safety and medical breakthroughs to be introduced to the health care markets. Cell-based product usage in the United Sates must be reported to the FDA.

With increasing complexity in cell sources, manipulations, and engineering processes, the potential harm to recipients is increased and therefore more scrutiny and regulation are necessary for patient safety. A brief review of milestone legislation provides a better understanding of the current regulations and may help foretell the direction of future safety rules.

The Biologics Control Act of 1902 was the first regulation intended to address the safety of emerging biologic products, such as vaccines. The act addressed the unintended introduction of tetanus via vaccines that at the time were produced in horses.[5] The 1902 act was updated and strengthened with passage of the 1906 Pure Food and Drug Act. This act empowered the federal government to oversee labeling of food and drug products. The power to write regulations and enforce them was granted to the agency that eventually became the FDA.[6] The Pure Food and Drug Act was updated through the Food, Drug, and Cosmetic Act of 1938 and provided the Secretary of Health and Human Services the authority to "promulgate regulations for the efficient enforcement" of the law.[7] In 1944, the Public Health Service Act (PHS Act) reconfirmed FDA oversight of biologic products used to treat or prevent disease.[8] The FDA is responsible for 2 directives:

1. Protecting the public health by assuring the safety, efficacy, and security of human drugs, biologic products, and medical devices
2. Advancing the public health by helping to speed innovations that make medicines more effective, safe, and affordable

They have a legal duty to review and approve the licensure application of drugs and devices intended to be marketed for human and veterinarian use.

The PHS Act also provides legal authority to the FDA to establish regulatory requirements for marketing human cells, tissues, and cellular and tissue-based products (HCT/Ps) and other biologic products derived from human cells that exceed the definition of HCT/Ps as found in 21 CFR 1271.10. The current PHS Act has 2 major sections of concern for cell therapy: Section 351 and Section 361. Section 351 identifies the characteristics of biologic products that must follow a path to licensure and introduces concepts of current good manufacturing practices (cGMPs), whereas Section 361 solely focuses on the need to prevent the introduction, transmission, and spread of communicable disease. Licensure is not required for 361 products but FDA registration of these activities with cell-based products is mandated.

Until around 2001, the approach to regulating HCT/Ps was highly fragmented. In 1993, the FDA introduced a new regulatory concept, through an interim rule, that required the distributors of human cells intended to treat or prevent disease in humans to implement a process to screen for risks of communicable disease, test for transmissible diseases, and maintain records of these activities.

In 1997, the FDA proposed a new approach to the regulation of HCT/Ps, seeking to establish a comprehensive oversight program. In accordance with the tiered risk-based approach, some HCT/Ps would be subject solely to regulations in Section 361 of the PHS Act (42 U.S.C. 264), whereas others would still be regulated as drugs, devices, and/or biologic products under the existing Section 351 (42 U.S.C. 262) and the Federal Food, Drug, and Cosmetic Act.

Provisions for 361 and 351 product regulations became effective in 2 stages. First, in April 2001, establishments whose products were already previously regulated under Section 361 were required to register their activities and implement policies to prevent introduction and spread of disease. Second, all manufacturers of cellular HCT/Ps (351 regulated products) were required to register their activities by January 2004, except if these products were being distributed under an investigational new drug/device (IND). In addition, as of May 25, 2005, manufacturers of HCT/Ps were required to comply with the current core good tissue practices, the other parts of 21 CFR 1271, and applicable regulations found within the same chapter.

Cellular biologic products are regulated as either HCT/Ps or biologic drugs products as defined in 21 CFR 1271.10. The distinction between product classifications is based on the risks associated with:

- The spread of disease from the donor source
- The intended function of the infused cells
- The potential for introducing contamination or cross contamination
- Undetected product mix-ups in the manufacturing processes

Products that do not meet all 4 elements are deemed to be biologic drug products.[9]

The regulations for manufacturing, storing, labeling, and distribution of these biologic drugs are found in the requirements for pharmaceutical drug manufacturing in 21 CFR 210 and 211 and biologic product manufacturing in 21 CFR 610. Manufacturers must follow all regulations applicable to their products from donor qualification to final distribution and may request assistance from the FDA through the Tissue Reference Group with determining the classification and regulatory pathway for the product under consideration.[10]

More advanced manipulations and manufacturing protocols for creating biologically active and sustained therapeutic effector cell drug products are most often in an investigational stage. These products are carefully studied for efficacy and safety as part of a plan to eventually license these drugs. Under 21 CFR 1271 and PHS Act Section 351, only licensed biologics drugs can be prescribed and distributed for infusion to patients. The use of unlicensed manipulated cells is allowed using protocols approved by a human subjects protection panel, such as an institutional review board , and receipt of safe-to-proceed notification from the FDA on their approval of the IND application for the defined indications or treatments. These INDs are reviewed by FDA scientists from the Center for Biologics Evaluation and Research with expertise in product chemistry, manufacturing, and controls (CMCs) as well as preclinical testing and clinical trial design for cell therapeutics.

To ensure the safety of these drug products, the manufacture is also required to comply with the cGMPs, which are found in 21 CFR 210, 211, and 610. A manufacturer should be planning for the submission of a biologics license application (BLA) that shows full cGMP compliance along with data generated from phase I, II, and III IND studies supporting the labeling claims for specific disease indications in order for the FDA to permit marketing of the drug as an approved therapy.

Cell-based products have been licensed by the FDA as drug products, whereas many others remain the subject of clinical trials intended to show safety and efficacy.

The recent licensure of 2 CAR T-cell products has stimulated clinical researchers to further pursue developing other therapies that may also eventually be licensed. Large pharmaceutical companies are now investing extensive resources in hopes of developing a licensed product that yields a substantial financial return. Successful licensure and potential financial gains are driving rapid advancements in cellular therapies.

MANAGING EMERGING INFORMATION, RISKS, AND EXPECTATIONS

There are 2 major regulatory document types that are applicable:

1. The rule or regulation
2. Any guidance for compliance as suggested by the FDA

Regulations are proposed by either presidential authority or congressional act in response to a threat to public health or to address a health concern. Federal regulations also require that an agency, such as the FDA, be granted authority to develop and enforce new or changed rules. Using the Federal Register (FR) as the recognized announcement vehicle, the agency is required to publish its authority to issue a new rule along with either a call for suggestions to address an identified issue or, more commonly, a draft of the proposed rule. The public, especially those to be regulated by the proposed rule, are invited to submit comments or suggest edits, which are addressed by a response publication in the FR. After the resolution of comments and review by lawyers to ensure that the measure does not exceed the agency's authority, the final rule is published with a date for expected implementation and compliance.

The agency publishes suggested compliance methods, as guidance, that align with the final rule. These guidance documents are usually described as the current thinking by both the FDA and industry. The FDA uses a very structured program, current good guidance practices, for the development, evaluation, and final publication of guidance documents. The process follows the same path as the implementation of new rules. The agency:

- Publishes a draft version
- Seeks comments
- Evaluates and addresses all comments

Industry comments often reshape the final guidance document. Although these guidance documents are not legally binding, manufacturers are responsible for providing evidence of substantial equivalence or a superior approach that complies with the final rule requirements (**Table 1**).[11,12]

New concepts and early promising results from cell-based products that exceed the definition of HCT/Ps need careful consideration and safety controls before extending biologic products for human use beyond bench research. Experience gained and lessons learned from safety studies, validation and verification exercises, and results from scaled-up manufacturing help shape strategies and/or control mechanisms that mitigate identified risks. Manipulations at the cellular level may generate unwanted consequences or unintended and unrepairable outcomes. These higher-risk products must be cautiously used in carefully designed clinical trials to determine efficacy, safety, and practical uses. The summary of the risk assessment, results from safety (animal) models, CMCs, and standard operating procedures (SOPs), at minimum in draft, are part of the IND submission. The agency may pose several questions or ask for more data in order to complete its safety review and risk/benefit analysis. When all safety concerns have been addressed and the safe-to-proceed letter is received, the clinical trial may begin treating patents.

Table 1
United States Food and Drug Administration guidance documents for human cells and tissues and cellular and gene therapy

Guidance Subject	Issue Date
1. CMCs for human GT INDs** Chemistry, Manufacturing, and Control (CMC) Information for Human Gene Therapy Investigational New Drug Applications (INDs); Draft Guidance for Industry	July 2018
2. Long-term follow-up after GT** Long Term Follow-up After Administration of Human Gene Therapy Products; Draft Guidance for Industry	July 2018
3. Testing of retroviral-based gene therapy for replication competent retrovirus** Testing of Retroviral Vector-Based Human Gene Therapy Products for Replication Competent Retrovirus During Product Manufacture and Patient Follow-up; Draft Guidance for Industry	July 2018
4. Gene therapy for hemophilia** Human Gene Therapy for Hemophilia; Draft Guidance for Industry	July 2018
5. Human gene therapy for rare diseases** Human Gene Therapy for Rare Diseases; Draft Guidance for Industry	July 2018
6. Human Gene Therapy for Retinal Disorders** Human Gene Therapy for Retinal Disorders; Draft Guidance for Industry	July 2018
7. Reducing Zika transmission risks* Donor Screening Recommendations to Reduce the Risk of Transmission of Zika Virus by Human Cells, Tissues, and Cellular and Tissue-Based Products; Guidance for Industry	May 2018, March 2016
8. Minimal manipulation and homologous use for HCTPs* Regulatory Considerations for Human Cells, Tissues, and Cellular and Tissue-Based Products: Minimal Manipulation and Homologous Use; Guidance for Industry and Food and Drug Administration Staff	December 2017
9. Same surgical procedure* Same Surgical Procedure Exception under 21 CFR 1271.15(b): Questions and Answers Regarding the Scope of the Exception; Guidance for Industry	November 2017
10. Evaluation of devices used in regenerative medicine** Evaluation of Devices Used with Regenerative Medicine Advanced Therapies; Draft Guidance for Industry	November 2017
11. Expedited review pathways for regenerative medicine therapies** Expedited Programs for Regenerative Medicine Therapies for Serious Conditions; Draft Guidance for Industry	November 2017
12. HCTP deviation reporting* Deviation Reporting for Human Cells, Tissues, and Cellular and Tissue-Based Products Regulated Solely Under Section 361 of the Public Health Service Act and 21 CFR Part 1271; Guidance for Industry	November 2017

(continued on next page)

Table 1 (continued)	
13. Nucleic acid tests for West Nile virus* Use of Nucleic Acid Tests to Reduce the Risk of Transmission of West Nile Virus from Living Donors of Human Cells, Tissues, and Cellular and Tissue-Based Product s (HCT/Ps); Guidance for Industry	May 2017, September 2016, December 2015
14. Donor eligibility: human-derived clotting factors* Revised Recommendations for Determining Eligibility of Donors of Human Cells, Tissues, and Cellular and Tissue-Based Products Who Have Received Human-Derived Clotting Factor Concentrates; Guidance for Industry	November 2016
15. Microbial vectors in gene therapy** Recommendations for Microbial Vectors Used for Gene Therapy; Guidance for Industry	September 2016
16. Nucleic acid tests for hepatitis B* Use of Nucleic Acid Tests to Reduce the Risk of Transmission of Hepatitis B Virus from Donors of Human Cells, Tissues, and Cellular and Tissue-Based Products; Guidance for Industry	August 2016
17. Reporting adverse reactions to HCTPs: 361 products* Investigating and Reporting Adverse Reactions Related to Human Cells, Tissues, and Cellular and Tissue-Based Products (HCT/Ps) Regulated Solely under Section 361 of the Public Health Service Act and 21 CFR Part 1271 - Guidance for Industry	March 2016
18. HCTP donor screening tests for *Treponema pallidum** Use of Donor Screening Tests to Test Donors of Human Cells, Tissues and Cellular and Tissue-Based Products for Infection with Treponema pallidum (Syphilis); Guidance for Industry	September 2015
19. Design and analysis of shedding studies for bacteria or viruses in gene therapy** Design and Analysis of Shedding Studies for Virus or Bacteria-Based Gene Therapy and Oncolytic Products; Guidance for Industry	August 2015
20. Early phase cell and gene therapy trials** Considerations for the Design of Early-Phase Clinical Trials of Cellular and Gene Therapy Products; Guidance for Industry	June 2015
21. Content of environmental assessments for gene therapy, vectored vaccines and recombinant viral and microbial products** Determining the Need for and Content of Environmental Assessments for Gene Therapies, Vectored Vaccines, and Related Recombinant Viral or Microbial Products; Guidance for Industry	March 2015
22. Biologics applications for cord blood for hematopoietic and immunologic reconstitution** Guidance for Industry: BLA for Minimally Manipulated, Unrelated Allogeneic Placental/Umbilical Cord Blood Intended for Hematopoietic and Immunologic Reconstitution in Patients with Disorders Affecting the Hematopoietic System	March 2014

(continued on next page)

Table 1
(continued)

23. INDs for cord blood for hematopoietic and immunologic reconstitution** IND Applications for Minimally Manipulated, Unrelated Allogeneic Placental/Umbilical Cord Blood Intended for Hematopoietic and Immunologic Reconstitution in Patients with Disorders Affecting the Hematopoietic System - Guidance for Industry and FDA Staff	March 2014
24. Preclinical assessments for investigational cellular and gene therapy products** Guidance for Industry: Preclinical Assessment of Investigational Cellular and Gene Therapy Products	November 2013
25. Current good tissue practices* Guidance for Industry: Current Good Tissue Practice (CGTP) and Additional Requirements for Manufacturers of Human Cells, Tissues, and Cellular and Tissue-Based Products (HCT/Ps)	December 2011
26. Preparing IDE and IND applications for knee cartilage** Guidance for Industry: Preparation of IDEs and INDs for Products Intended to Repair or Replace Knee Cartilage	December 2011, 2007
27. Therapeutic cancer vaccines** Guidance for Industry: Clinical Considerations for Therapeutic Cancer Vaccines	October 2011
28. Class II controls for cord blood processing systems and storage containers* Guidance for Industry: Class II Special Controls Guidance Document: Cord Blood Processing System and Storage Container	March 2011
29. Potency tests for cell and gene therapies** Guidance for Industry: Potency Tests for Cellular and Gene Therapy Products	January 2011, October 2008
30. Cell therapy for cardiac disease** Guidance for Industry: Cellular Therapy for Cardiac Disease	October 2010
31. Allogeneic pancreatic islet cells** Guidance for Industry: Considerations for Allogeneic Pancreatic Islet Cell Products	September 2009
32. Guidance for reviewers and sponsors of cell and gene therapy INDs** Guidance for FDA Reviewers and Sponsors: Content and Review of Chemistry, Manufacturing, and Control (CMC) Information for Human Gene Therapy Investigational New Drug Applications (INDs)	April 2008
33. Guidance for reviewers and sponsors of somatic cell INDs** Guidance for FDA Reviewers and Sponsors: Content and Review of Chemistry, Manufacturing, and Control (CMC) Information for Human Somatic Cell Therapy Investigational New Drug Applications (INDs)	April 2008
34. Donor testing using pooled specimens for communicable disease testing* Guidance for Industry: Certain Human Cells, Tissues, and Cellular and Tissue-Based Products (HCT/Ps) Recovered from Donors Who Were Tested for Communicable Diseases Using Pooled Specimens or Diagnostic Tests	April 2008

(continued on next page)

Table 1 *(continued)*	
35. Small entity HCTP compliance guide* Regulation of Human Cells, Tissues, and Cellular and Tissue-Based Products (HCT/Ps) - Small Entity Compliance Guide; Guidance for Industry	August 2007
36. Eligibility determination* Eligibility Determination for Donors of Human Cells, Tissues, and Cellular and Tissue-Based Products; Guidance for Industry	August 2007
37. Delayed reactions in cell and GT trials** Guidance for Industry: Gene Therapy Clinical Trials - Observing Subjects for Delayed Adverse Events	November 2006
38. Testing for replication competent retrovirus** Guidance for Industry; Supplemental Guidance on Testing for Replication Competent Retrovirus in Retroviral Vector Based Gene Therapy Products and During Follow-up of Patients in Clinical Trials Using Retroviral Vectors	November 2006
39. Manufacturing agreements* Guidance for Industry: Compliance with 21 CFR Part 1271. 150(c)(1) – Manufacturing Arrangements	September 2006
40. Labeling claim for screening tests using cadaveric samples* Guidance for Industry: Recommendations for Obtaining a Labeling Claim for Communicable Disease Donor Screening Tests Using Cadaveric Blood Specimens from Donors of Human Cells, Tissues, and Cellular and Tissue-Based Products (HCT/Ps)	June 2000
41. Validation of procedures to process tissues* Guidance for Industry: Validation of Procedures for Processing of Human Tissues Intended for Transplantation	March 2002
42. Availability of licensed donor screening tests for cadaveric specimens* Availability of Licensed Donor Screening Tests Labeled for Use with Cadaveric Blood Specimens; Guidance for Industry	June 2000
43. Guidance for somatic cell and gene therapies** Guidance for Industry: Guidance for Human Somatic Cell Therapy and Gene Therapy	March 1998
44. Screening and testing tissues for transplant* Guidance for Industry: Screening and Testing of Donors of Human Tissue Intended for Transplantation	July 1997

* HCT/P tissue guidance; ** Cellular and GT guidance.

Data from U.S. Food and Drug Administration (FDA). Tissue Guidances. Available at: https://www.fda.gov/vaccines-blood-biologics/biologics-guidances/tissue-guidances. Accessed May 20 2019; and U.S. Food and Drug Administration (FDA). Vaccine and Related Biological Product Guidances. Available at: https://www.fda.gov/vaccines-blood-biologics/biologics-guidances/vaccine-and-related-biological-product-guidances. Accessed May 20 2019.

On completion of the trial, clinical data coupled with the validation data generated from the manufacturing runs, using approved SOPs and policies, is statistically evaluated for outcomes, robustness, and power to establish human safety and efficacy claims. These data form the basis for the FDA's decision regarding approval or denial of the BLA.

The FDA uses the term postmarketing commitments (PMCs) to refer to an agreement by the investigator to conduct additional specified studies as part of the approval of the IND or licensure application.[13] These studies are designed to monitor the safety, efficacy, and/or optimal use of the product and ensure consistency and reliability of product quality. Before the passage of newer regulations, the FDA could only require PMCs in cases of accelerated approvals or for studies that were required to show clinical benefit. The Food and Drug Administration Modernization Act of 1997 (the Modernization Act) added a new provision requiring PMCs for biologic products, opening this option for products that may meet unmet therapeutic needs.

The Modernization Act requires reporting of additional safety information, including data about a serious risk or an unexpected serious adverse event related to the use of the drug. Even if a serious risk is known at the time of drug approval, postapproval studies may provide additional data about frequency or severity of adverse events that is new safety information. This same act gives FDA the authority to require a risk evaluation and mitigation strategy (REMS) from manufacturers to ensure that the benefits of a drug or biologic product continue to outweigh its risks.[14]

A REMS may be required by the FDA as part of the approval of a new product or when new safety concerns about an approved product are identified. A REMS plan is a safety strategy to manage known or potential serious risks associated with these biologic drugs but still allow access for patients when the benefit may outweigh the risk.

INDUSTRY STANDARDS AND ACCREDITATION

Balancing the wealth of available cell biology knowledge and new discoveries that may provide care to critically ill patients with urgent medical needs against regulations, policies, and guidance documents for developing safe, stable, and reproducible medical products without stifling medical breakthroughs and innovations is overwhelming.

The cellular therapy field has 2 industry facilitated accrediting bodies with published requirements that are developed by qualified member volunteers who use their knowledge and experience to establish consensus for practice standards. These organizations are the AABB and the Foundation for the Accreditation of Cellular Therapy (FACT). In 1991, AABB first incorporated cell therapy accreditation standards within the 14th edition of *Standards for Blood Banks and Transfusion Services*. These early standards focused on quality systems, donor screening, product collections, and laboratory processing. Five years later, AABB published its first edition of *Standards for Hematopoietic Progenitor Cells*, shifting these standards into a stand-alone document and away from the *Standards for Blood Banks and Transfusion Services*. AABB consolidated and merged standards in 2004 from different cell sources, the 2001 *Cord Blood Standards* and the *Standards for Hematopoietic Progenitor Cells* to create the first edition of the *Cellular Therapy Product Services Standards*. In 2013, AABB expanded the 13th edition of the *Cellular Therapy Product Services Standards* to include clinical care activities (**Table 2**)[15]. FACT issued its first edition of standards in 1996 and accredited the first program in 1998. Since this first hematopoietic cellular therapy edition, FACT has developed separate and stand-alone accreditation standards for cord blood banks (currently sixth edition July 2016), common standards for cellular therapies (first edition March 2015, second edition 2019), and immune effector cells (first edition January 2017) (**Table 3**)[16]. AABB and FACT have short histories in standards setting and accrediting member facilities for cellular therapy activities but both leverage the expertise and experience of their members to shape new editions of standards that are also internationally adopted.

Table 2 American Association of Blood Banks: history of cellular therapy standards and accreditation	
Year	Activity
1991	The 14th edition of blood bank transfusion service standards included standards for collection, storage and distribution of human cells for transplant and bone marrow products
1996	The first edition of HPCs standards was published
2001	The first edition of CB standards was published
2004	The HPC and CB standards were merged to create the first edition of the CT standards
2013	Standards for clinical practice activities were added to the sixth edition of the CT standards

Abbreviations: CB, cord blood; CT, cellular therapy; HPC, hematopoietic progenitor cell.
Data from AABB. Standards programs history. Available at: http://www.aabb.org/sa/standards/Documents/standards-programs-history.pdf. Accessed on Jan 12 2019.

FUTURE DIRECTIONS

Reports of successful early-phase trials have generated an expansion of new and innovative ideas and applications for stem cells. The rapid exchange of peer-reviewed articles, the ease of travel for presentations at national and international scientific and medical conferences, and increased collaborations between institutions has led to exponential growth in the development of novel investigational products. Reported and promoted uses of cellular therapies for treating a variety of maladies has sparked increased interest via social media outlets. This access to information in the public domain has created a desire by patients to seek out any treatment they can afford. Patients feel more comfortable approaching a physician with the hope that they can potentially receive cell-based products. Social media networks are easily accessed forums by laypersons who can quickly find advertising promotions of often unproven cellular therapies. These unregulated and uncontrolled medical services may cause more harm than benefit to the patients.

For scientifically sound and ethical treatment, the public and medical community need to understand the differences between clinical trials of investigational drug products and medical treatment innovations. Clinical trials involve controlled studies that collect data using methods to minimize bias and answer questions about safety and efficacy. Data are evaluated to determine benefit to future patient populations. These results are published to inform the greater medical community. These volunteer human subjects are protected by policies and procedures developed by the National Institutes of Health and the FDA. Compliance with these procedures and policies helps to ensure that other volunteers are willing to participate in future trials.

Medically innovative products or treatments may be viewed as ethical and legitimate uses of nonapproved therapies by qualified professionals within their practice of medicine and scope of their licenses. These treatments are intended to only benefit specific patients. The recognition of the differences between investigational studies and individualized treatment plans benefits both the medical community and general populations.

Over the last couple of decades, major advancements in medical applications of cellular therapy and cell biology have occurred. This upsurge in cell therapy clinical investigations has led to exciting innovations in patient care with an extremely broad range of applications in numerous diseases. However, initial experiments and clinical trials have also revealed unanticipated risks that needed mitigation before safely

Table 3
Timeline of major achievements

Year	Achievements
Founding of FACT	
1992	ASBMT Clinical Affairs Committee developed the first Clinical Standards for Hematopoietic Cell Transplantation. Parent organization International Society for Hematotherapy and Graft Engineering (ISHAGE) formed. (Currently named International Society Cell & Gene Therapy [ISCT].)
1993	Parent organization American Society for Blood and Marrow Transplantation (ASBMT) formed. (Currently named American Society for Transplantation and Cellular Therapy [ASTCT].) Regulatory Affairs Committee of ISHAGE developed first draft of laboratory standards for Hematopoietic Cell Collection and Processing.
1994	ASBMT Clinical Standards for Hematopoietic Cell Transplantation and ISHAGE laboratory Standards for Hematopoietic Cell Collection and Processing merged into a single document. North American Task Force (NATF) concluded that FACT Standards were of sufficiently high quality to serve as a template for the other organizations involved in this field.
1995	Co-founded by ASBMT and ISCT, the Foundation for the Accreditation of Hematopoietic Cell Therapy (FAHCT) was formed for the purpose of: 1. Establishing standards for quality medical and laboratory practice 2. Implementing voluntary inspection and accreditation program
FACT Pivotal Events	
1996	First edition of FAHCT Standards for Hematopoietic Progenitor Cell Collection, Processing & Transplantation published.
1997	Inspection and Accreditation program began.
1998	First cell therapy transplant programs awarded FAHCT accreditation.
1999	FAHCT Standards adopted by JACIE (Joint Accreditation Committee EBMT-ISCT).
2000	FAHCT and NetCord partnered to develop international standards for cord blood collection, processing, testing, banking, selection, and release.
2001	Name changed to the Foundation for the Accreditation of Cellular Therapy (FACT) to encompass, in addition to hematopoietic cell products and therapies, new and exciting therapies such as those using mesenchymal stem cells, dendritic cells, targeted lymphocytes, genetically modified cells, pancreatic islets, and others.
2002	Second Edition of FACT Cellular Therapy Standards published. Cord Blood Bank Inspection and Accreditation program began.
2006	FACT celebrated its 10th anniversary. Third Edition of Cellular Therapy Standards developed and published jointly by FACT and JACIE. Third Edition of Cord Blood Standards developed and published jointly by FACT and NetCord.
2007	FACT committee structure established to lead the organization's strategic initiatives. FACT accreditation added to methodology to determine the U.S. News & World report rankings of transplant centers for the "America's Best Hospitals" and "America's Best Children's Hospitals" lists.

(*continued on next page*)

Table 3 (continued)	
Year	Achievements
2008	Educational efforts expanded to include online webinars and tutorials. Fourth Edition of FACT-JACIE Cellular Therapy Standards published.
2010	Fourth Edition of NetCord-FACT Cord Blood Standards published.
2012	Fifth Edition of FACT-JACIE Cellular Therapy Standards published. FACTWeb online accreditation portal launched. Accreditation of laboratories performing more-than-minimal manipulation began. FACT accredited first cell therapy programs in Brazil and Asia.
2013	Fifth Edition of NetCord-FACT Cord Blood Standards published. New Task Forces launched – Clinical Outcomes, Data Management, and Payer Relations. FACT Consulting Services piloted to assist transplant centers. FACT accredited first cord blood banks in Greece and Hong Kong.
2014	FACT accredited first cord blood bank in Brazil. FACT accredited first private cord blood bank in the United States.
2015	Sixth Edition of FACT-JACIE Cellular Therapy Standards published. First Edition of FACT Common Standards for Cellular Therapies published. FACT accredited first cord blood banks in Saudi Arabia and Turkey. FACT Consulting Services officially launched.
2016	FACT celebrated its 20th anniversary. FACT began formally reviewing clinical outcomes. Sixth Edition of NetCord-FACT Cord Blood Standards published. FACT accredited first cell therapy program in Mexico. FACT accredited first cord blood banks in India and Cyprus.
2017	First Edition of FACT Standards for Immune Effector Cells published. FACT and Center for International Blood and Marrow Transplant Research (CIBMTR) began collaborative data audit program. FACT accredited first cord blood bank in Portugal.
2018	Seventh Edition of FACT-JACIE Cellular Therapy Standards published. FACT and the Sociedade Brasileira de Transplante de Medula Óssea (SBTMO) announced formal partnership to develop joint FACT-SBTMO Cellular Therapy Accreditation Program in Brazil. New FACT accreditation portal launched.
2019	Second Edition of FACT Common Standards for Cellular Therapies published.

From The Foundation for the Accreditation of Cellular Therapy at the University of Nebraska Medical Center. Timeline of major achievements. Available at: http://www.factwebsite.org/About_FACT/Major_Achievements.aspx. Accessed July 10 2019; with permission.

proceeding, especially regarding the impact of cell-based therapeutic approaches for the risk of cancer development and unintended malignant transformation. Both the scientific and medical communities are now aware of these problems and limitations, and the challenges that lie ahead have now been identified. Current investigations and new approaches based on recent advances in the biological understanding of mechanisms controlling stem cell fate are improving the tools and strategies that influence clinical outcome.

As these developments and documented successes from controlled clinical trials are published, scientists are inspired to investigate possible modifications for better or sustained outcomes. Novel products and new clinical trials are gaining approvals, and a balance between regulated safety controls and the desire to try these products in human patients must be achieved. The FDA is approving more IND applications for clinical trials but it is also beginning to require robust PMCs, which balances the need to make these life-changing therapies available but also provides the responsible authorities with the necessary data to determine a level of confidence in the safety and efficacy of these products.

As the demand for robust and sound data for rapid decision making escalates, there is an anticipated need for increased international collaboration for harmonization of regulatory mechanisms that require safety and efficacy reporting in peer-reviewed literature. Data integrity regulations will be a focus in the near future. Data for critical decision making have integrity when it is complete, consistent, and accurate.[17] All clinical trial sponsors and licensed product holders should recognize the need to design data management systems to meet requirements for data collection that is ALCOA:

- Attributable to the person generating it
- Legible to assure interpretation
- Contemporaneous or concurrently recorded
- Original
- Accurate

Standardized international requirements, such as International Council on Harmonisation (ICH) Q7, call for the design of processes for generation, retention, and compliance verification of data integrity found in the ALCOA requirements. Successful implementation and maintenance of ICH Q7 requirements may provide reviewers and decisions makers with the assurances needed to use that information to expedite health care approaches and drug product licensures. Shared data from clinical trials or PMCs that follow ALCOA requirements will most likely become sources of information for international regulators.

Innovation and breakthrough will be balanced with standardization of acceptable safety practices. National Health Authority regulators, such as the FDA, Health Canada, European Medicines Agency, and Swiss Medic, play a vital role in the development of sound legislation and provide interpretation, guidance, and education. Industry self-regulation through voluntary accreditation processes will also have an increased presence as a driving force for developing practice standards to rapidly but safely deliver novel biologic drug products and identify potential risks associated with emerging therapies.

A recent development that will quickly advance delivery of cellular therapy medicines is the 21st Century Cures Act,[18] which provides 4 paths to expedited approval of an IND or licensure. The accelerated paths are designated as:

1. Fast track
2. Breakthrough therapy
3. Accelerated approval
4. Priority review

For a biologic drug product to be designated into one of these 4 paths, it must meet at least 1 of the following:

1. Address a serious condition
2. Be similar to an available therapy
3. Address an unmet need

Intended to assist industry in determining the most appropriate regulatory pathway, the FDA published the *Guidance for Industry: Expedited Programs for Regenerative*

Medicine Therapies for Serious Conditions, which defines criteria needed to seek an expedited designation as:

1. Fast track
2. Breakthrough therapy
3. Regenerative medicine advanced therapy (RMAT)[19]

Regenerative medicine is an approach that has great potential to treat serious medical conditions. The FDA has determined that a biologic cell-based drug product regulated as a 351 HCT/P may be considered for designation as an RMAT product.[20] Therefore, IND-governed products will be considered for breakthrough or fast-track designation under the 21st Centuries Cure Act. Manufacturers can expect faster approvals of their INDs and licensure applications.

Accelerated approvals of more licensed, cell-based therapies will require a shift in practices and standards toward requiring implementation of cGMP requirements. cGMP approaches will be applied to activities such as:

- Qualifying donors and determining suitability and eligibility
- Qualifying vendors and suppliers of critical materials through on-site inspections
- Increasing specifications for practices that mitigate the risks of contamination, cross contamination or mix-ups
- Standardizing requirements for approval of the release of products for labeling and distribution

Current documentation and record-keeping practices need to be revised to meet the cGMPs, good documentation practices, and ALCOA expectations to show evidence of reproducible manufacturing procedures, supporting the claim of safe products for human use. These practices will provide the medical community with increased confidence that rapid developments in cellular therapy can safely be introduced into the clinical setting.

The key to safely developing and introducing biologic drug products into mainstream patient care is a harmonized approach within countries and internationally. The fastest route for the introduction of these products and practices is integration of regulations with industry-developed practice standards. Informed industry members will drive the direction of rules, regulations, guidance, and standards by actively voicing their opinions and concerns during comment periods. Collaborative efforts between regulators, manufacturers, and clinicians to create a sustainable regulatory framework will provide the shortest path to the delivery and marketing of safe and reliable cell-based biologic drug products to patients.

REFERENCES

1. Pillow RP, Epstein RB, Buckner CD, et al. Treatment of bone-marrow failure by isogeneic marrow infusion. N Engl J Med 1966;275:94–7.
2. Gatti RA, Meuwissen HJ, Allen HD, et al. Immunological reconstitution of sex-linked lymphopenic immunological deficiency. Lancet 1968;292:1366–9.
3. Kim D, Kim C-H, Moon J, et al. Generation of human induced pluripotent stem cells by direct delivery of reprogramming proteins. Cell Stem Cell 2009;4: 472–6.
4. Chu VT, Weber T, Wefers B, et al. Increasing the efficiency of homology-directed repair for CRISPR- Cas-9- induced precise gene editing in mammalian cells. Nat Biotechnol 2015;33:543–8.

5. Harden VA. A short history of the National Institutes of Health. Available at: https://history.nih.gov/exhibits/history/docs/page_03.html. Accessed March 13, 2019.
6. Carpenter DP. Pure food and drug act (1906) Major Acts of Congress. Available at: https://www.encyclopedia.com. Accessed March 13, 2019.
7. Federal food, drug and cosmetic act of 1938. Available at: https://ballotpedia.org/Federal_Food,_Drug,_and_Cosmetic_Act_of_1938. Accessed March 13, 2019.
8. Public Health Service Act, 1944. Public health reports 1974: 468. Available at: https://www.ncbi.nlm.nih.gov/pmc/articles/PMC1403520/pdf/pubhealthrep00059-0006. Accessed March 13, 2019.
9. Frequently asked questions about therapeutic biological products. Available at: https://wwwut.fda.gov/Drugs/DevelopmentApprovalProcess/HowDrugsareDevelopedandApproved/ApprovalApplications/TherapeuticBiologicApplications/ucm113522.htm. Accessed March 13, 2019.
10. Tissue reference group. Available at: https://www.fda.gov/BiologicsBloodVaccines/TissueTissueProducts/RegulationofTissues/ucm152857.htm. Accessed March 13, 2019.
11. U.S. Food and Drug Administration (FDA). Tissue guidances. Available at: https://www.fda.gov/vaccines-blood-biologics/biologics-guidances/tissue-guidances. Accessed May 20, 2019.
12. U.S. Food and Drug Administration (FDA). Vaccine and related biological product guidances. Available at: https://www.fda.gov/vaccines-blood-biologics/biologics-guidances/vaccine-and-related-biological-product-guidances. Accessed May 20, 2019.
13. Postmarketing requirements and commitments: legislative background. Available at: https://www.fda.gov/Drugs/GuidanceComplianceRegulatoryInformation/Post-marketingPhaseIVCommitments/ucm064633.htm. Accessed March 13, 2019.
14. Risk evaluation and mitigation strategies (REMS). Available at: https://www.fda.gov/Drugs/DrugSafety/REMS/default.htm. Accessed March 13, 2019.
15. Standards programs history. Available at: http://www.aabb.org/sa/standards/Documents/standards-programs-history.pdf. Accessed January 12, 2019.
16. The Foundation for the accreditation of cellular therapy at the University of Nebraska Medical Center. Timeline of major achievements. Available at: http://www.factwebsite.org/About_FACT/Major_Achievements.aspx. Accessed January 12, 2019.
17. Guidance for industry: data integrity and compliance with drug cgmp questions and answers. Available at: https://www.fda.gov/downloads/drugs/guidances/ucm495891.pdf. Accessed March 14, 2019.
18. 21st century cures ACT. Available at: https://www.congress.gov/114/bills/hr34/BILLS-114hr34enr.pdf. Accessed March 14, 2019.
19. Guidance for industry: Expedited Programs for regenerative medicine therapies for serious conditions. Available at: https://www.fda.gov/downloads/BiologicsBloodVaccines/GuidanceComplianceRegulatoryInformation/Guidances/CellularandGeneTherapy/UCM585414.pdf. Accessed March 13, 2019.
20. Regenerative medicine advanced therapy determination. Available at: https://www.fda.gov/biologicsbloodvaccines/cellulargenetherapyproducts/ucm537670.htm. Accessed March 13. 2019.

Approaches to Bloodless Surgery for Oncology Patients

Steven M. Frank, MD[a],*, Shruti Chaturvedi, MBBS, MS[b],
Ruchika Goel, MD, MPH[c,d,e], Linda M.S. Resar, MD[f]

KEYWORDS

- Anemia • Blood conservation • Bloodless • Cancer • Oncology • Surgery

KEY POINTS

- Bloodless surgery means providing perioperative care to patients who cannot be transfused because of religious beliefs, personal reasons, or alloimmunization, whereby compatible blood cannot be obtained.
- Diagnosing preoperative anemia at least 4 weeks before surgery generally allows sufficient time to determine the cause and provide treatment, which should be individualized for each patient. For erythropoiesis-stimulating agents, the risks and benefits should be assessed for each individual patient.
- Intraoperative blood loss with cancer surgery can be reduced by meticulous surgical technique, topical hemostatic agents, hemostatic variations of electrocautery, maintaining normothermia, controlled hypotension, antifibrinolytic medications, and acute normovolemic hemodilution.

Continued

Disclosure: S.M. Frank has served on scientific advisory boards for Haemonetics, Medtronic, and Baxter. Each of these companies is involved with patient blood management. The other authors declare no conflicts of interest.
[a] Department of Anesthesiology/Critical Care Medicine, Center for Bloodless Medicine and Surgery, Johns Hopkins Health System Blood Management Clinical Community, The Armstrong Institute for Patient Safety and Quality, The Johns Hopkins Medical Institutions, Zayed 6208, 1800 Orleans Street, Baltimore, MD 21287, USA; [b] Division of Hematology, Department of Medicine, The Johns Hopkins Medical Institutions, Johns Hopkins Hospital, Ross Building Room 1032, 1800 Orleans Street, Baltimore, MD 21287, USA; [c] Division of Transfusion Medicine, Department of Pathology, The Johns Hopkins Medical Institutions, Baltimore, MD, USA; [d] Division of Hematology/Oncology, Simmons Cancer Institute at SIU School of Medicine, 315 West Carpenter Street, Springfield, IL 62702, USA; [e] Mississippi Valley Regional Blood Center; [f] Department of Medicine (Hematology), Oncology & Institute for Cellular Engineering, The Johns Hopkins Medical Institutions, Center for Bloodless Medicine and Surgery, Ross Building Room 1015, 1800 Orleans Street, Baltimore, MD 21287, USA
* Corresponding author.
E-mail address: sfrank3@jhmi.edu

Hematol Oncol Clin N Am 33 (2019) 857–871
https://doi.org/10.1016/j.hoc.2019.05.009
0889-8588/19/© 2019 Elsevier Inc. All rights reserved.

hemonc.theclinics.com

Continued

- Cell salvage in cancer surgery is controversial. The risk/benefit ratio should be considered for each case, and a leukoreduction filter may improve patient safety.
- Phlebotomy blood loss can be substantial, especially in intensive care units. Smaller tubes along with less frequent laboratory draws decrease the incidence and severity of hospital-acquired anemia.

INTRODUCTION

It has been said that there is no such thing as bloodless surgery; however, for 100 years, between the discovery of anesthesia in the 1840s and the advent of modern blood banking in the 1940s, surgery was bloodless by necessity. The average adult patient with a total blood volume of 5 L and a hemoglobin (Hb) concentration of 14 g/dL can afford to lose approximately 2.5 L (half their blood volume) before reaching the current recommended Hb threshold for transfusion (7 g/dL).[1] Cancer surgery has evolved, especially over the past 3 decades, with minimally invasive approaches such as laparoscopic and robotic procedures resulting in dramatically reduced blood loss and transfusion rates. The modern term, bloodless surgery, refers to perioperative care for patients who cannot be transfused, usually for religious or personal reasons, or for those with alloantibodies for whom compatible blood cannot be obtained. The focus of this article is on the clinical management of oncology patients who require or request bloodless surgery.

Modern bloodless surgery was first described by Ott and Cooley[2] in the 1970s, when they performed hundreds of cardiac surgeries on Jehovah's Witness (JW) patients who, according to their beliefs, would not accept allogeneic transfusions. The general population also began seeking bloodless care in the early 1980s, when the first transfusion-transmitted cases of human immunodeficiency (HIV) were reported. Although blood became safer in 1985 with HIV screening, and again in 1990 with hepatitis C screening, the general public was suddenly aware (and afraid) of transfusion-related risks. What followed was a series of 10 large, randomized clinical trials comparing lower with higher Hb transfusion thresholds, most of which have been published over the past decade, and all of which support the concept that "less is more," or what has been termed a restrictive transfusion strategy.[3,4] These studies are the evidence behind evidence-based transfusion practice, because 6 of the studies showed no benefit and 4 showed worse outcomes with the higher Hb threshold (a liberal transfusion strategy).[5] As a result, clinicians who were trained to keep the Hb level greater than 10 g/dL in the 1980s are now comfortable with a Hb transfusion trigger of 7 to 8 g/dL in patients who are not actively bleeding and hemodynamically stable.

Providing bloodless surgical care by no means implies simply withholding blood. Instead, a combination of methods are described in this article to achieve optimal blood conservation. The various methods are summarized in **Box 1**, and are categorized into those applicable to the preoperative, intraoperative, and postoperative periods. Clinical studies with propensity matching show that well-delivered bloodless care results in similar outcomes to those achieved in patients accepting transfusion. There were favorable results in both medical and surgical patients (**Fig. 1**),[6] and this type of specialized care was associated with 12% to 14% lower hospital costs and charges.[6] In a propensity matched analysis in a cardiac surgery study, there is evidence that bloodless patients had fewer acute complications, a shorter length of stay, and a reduced 1-year mortality.[7]

Box 1
Methods of blood conservation for bloodless surgical oncology patients

Preoperative

Early diagnosis and treatment of preoperative anemia[18]

Discontinuing herbal supplements that interfere with coagulation[26,27]

Discontinuing anticoagulants

Judicious decision making for when to not operate (risk exceeds benefit)

Intraoperative

Meticulous surgical technique

Intraoperative autologous blood salvage[41]

Intraoperative autologous normovolemic hemodilution[31]

Perioperative antifibrinolytics (tranexamic acid, epsilon aminocaproic acid)[32]

New methods of electrocautery[42]

Topical sealants and hemostatic agents[39]

Avoiding perioperative hypothermia[30]

Controlled hypotension

Point-of-care coagulation testing (viscoelastic testing)

Postoperative

Tolerating lower Hb levels[9,10,12]

Minimizing laboratory testing[15]

Low-volume Microtainers for phlebotomy

In-line blood-return devices for arterial and central venous catheters

Bloodless care shares many principles in common with patient blood management (PBM), which is intended to prevent and manage anemia, optimize coagulation to reduce or prevent hemorrhage, and promote optimal blood conservation, in order to improve outcomes using a patient-centric approach.[8] The primary difference is that PBM is intended to reduce unnecessary transfusions, whereas bloodless care is intended to avoid them altogether. The same general methods are used in both programs, and are reviewed in this article. In effect, bloodless care is simply extreme PBM.

JEHOVAH'S WITNESSES AND THEIR BELIEFS

It is important to understand the JWs' beliefs, because these patients make up most of the patients seeking bloodless care. The JW faith has more than 8 million members worldwide, with an estimated 1.2 million members in the United States. The avoidance of blood products has its origin in both the Old and New testaments of the Bible (Genesis 9:4, Leviticus 17:10–14, Acts 15:29, and Acts 21:25).[9] For example, in Leviticus 17:14 it is stated: "For the life of every sort of flesh is its blood, because the life is in it. Consequently, I state to the Israelites: You must not eat the blood of any sort of flesh, because the life of every sort of flesh is its blood." The prohibition of transfusion officially began in 1945 when doctrines were adopted that forbid the acceptance of blood products considered to be major fractions of blood, which include red blood

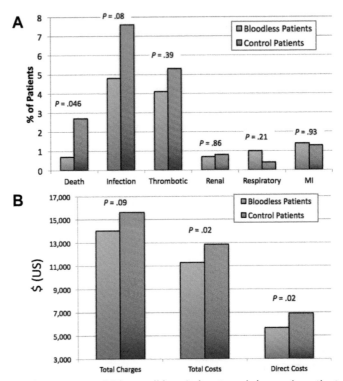

Fig. 1. (*A*) Clinical outcomes and (*B*) overall hospital costs and charges in patients receiving bloodless care compared with matched control patients who accept transfusion. Major morbidity was similar, with a trend toward fewer hospital-acquired infections, and in-hospital mortality was reduced in the bloodless patient group. Total hospital costs and charges were 12% to 14% less in the patients receiving bloodless care compared with those patients accepting transfusion. MI, myocardial infarction. (*Data from* Frank SM, Wick EC, Dezern AE, et al. Risk-adjusted clinical outcomes in patients enrolled in a bloodless program. Transfusion 2014;54(10 Pt 2):2668-77.)

cells, plasma, and platelets, as well as whole blood and white blood cells (**Fig. 2**).[10,11] In contrast, blood products and factors designated minor fractions are accepted by most JWs, although this is left to the discretion of the individual patient. Minor fractions include cryoprecipitate, individual clotting factors, prothrombin complex concentrate, immune globulin, and other blood-derived agents such as the thrombin-containing topical hemostatic agents. JWs also do not predonate autologous blood before surgery for later transfusion, because they believe that blood should not be separated from the body. Other blood-conserving methods that are acceptable to most JWs but a personal decision include autologous cell salvage, acute normovolemic hemodilution (ANH), as well as circuits that divert blood flow outside the body such as hemodialysis and cardiopulmonary bypass.

However, it is common for both JW patients and their medical care providers to be unfamiliar with the concepts of major and minor fractions of blood because these terms are not used by health care providers and blood banks. To avoid misunderstandings, many JW patients are encouraged by religious leaders to carry a wallet card listing advanced directives that specify blood components and blood conservation techniques that are acceptable and those that are not. The authors have often

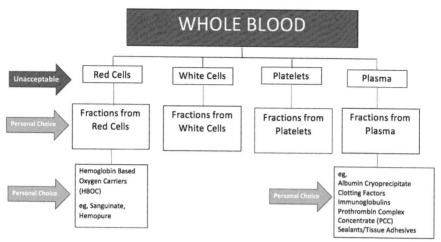

Fig. 2. Blood and blood components that are unacceptable or acceptable but by personal choice according to the JW Watchtower organization. JW patients do not accept what they call major fractions of blood (red blood cells, plasma, platelets, whole blood, and white blood cells). All other blood-derived components are referred to as minor fractions of blood, and these are considered acceptable, but by personal choice that must be made according to each patient's spiritual beliefs. (*Modified from* Watchtower ONLINE Library. Blood Fractions and Surgical Procedures. Available: at: https://wol.jw.org/en/wol/d/r1/lp-e/1102008086. Accessed Jan 12 2019; with permission.)

observed disagreements among family members at the bedside who may be more (or less) adamant about following religious doctrines. On occasion, elders from the church or hospital liaison committee members discusses options with the patients to help them make informed decisions. In the absence of these individuals, a bloodless program often has a coordinator who is a JW and can describe blood products in the context of their religious doctrines. In the setting of life-threatening anemia, the authors also try to confirm the patient's wishes in the absence of family members or members of the JW faith to help ensure that the patient does not feel pressured to avoid blood products. We have also cared for JW patients who decide to accept blood products as long as their wishes are not disclosed. The most important practical aspect of the preoperative visit is to complete the informed consent, and there are many variations of this type of document. When counseled by a knowledgeable team member, in our experience, more than 90% of JWs make the personal choice to accept all the minor fractions and other blood-conserving methods. JWs do not accept whole blood or leukocytes; however, these products are rarely administered in most hospitals.

THE PROVIDER CARE TEAM

In a well-established bloodless program, a team approach is used to provide optimal care. Members of the team include representatives from anesthesiology, hematology, surgery, transfusion medicine, nursing, critical care, and pharmacy. The bloodless coordinator often plays a critical role, particularly if that individual is a JW who can describe the blood products in the context of their religious beliefs. JW members of the team generally make patients and family members feel more comfortable with their care and options. For patients who cannot be transfused, it is paramount to diagnose anemia in advance of a planned surgery to ensure that anemia is treated, as detailed next.

PREOPERATIVE PREPARATION

The 2 primary goals of preoperative care are to diagnose and treat anemia, and discontinue any medications or herbal supplements that could worsen bleeding. Because bleeding disorders, such as von Willebrand disease, are common and can cause excessive surgical bleeding, the authors also screen patients for acquired or genetic bleeding dyscrasias. A challenge of managing preoperative anemia is obtaining laboratory results in time to diagnose and effectively treat the anemia. Some centers routinely order preoperative laboratory tests just 2 to 3 days before surgery, which precludes correction of the anemia before the surgery. There are 2 main considerations in determining the appropriate preoperative Hb target. The first is the expected blood loss for a given surgery, which is poorly understood among providers who are not involved with surgery. For example, many do not know that a typical thyroidectomy patient loses less than 50 mL of blood (about 1% of their total blood volume, or roughly 3 tablespoons) and thus there is no urgency in treating mild or even moderate preoperative anemia. For surgeries with minimal blood loss, a preoperative Hb target of only 8 to 10 g/dL is sufficient, and the cause and treatment of anemia can be managed after the surgery.

On the other end of the spectrum are surgeries associated with significant blood loss, such as cardiac surgery, in which the average decrease in Hb level postoperatively can range from 3 to 5 g/dL, even with optimal bloodless techniques. In such cases, the authors take into account the estimated blood volume based on body mass to calculate the blood loss that could be tolerated by each individual patient. For most adults, we estimate 70 mL/kg total blood volume, such that a smaller 40-kg patient has an estimated blood volume of only 2.8 L, whereas an 80-kg patient has an estimated blood volume of 5.6 L. Thus, the larger patient can generally lose twice as much blood as the smaller patient before a critically low Hb level is reached.[1,12]

A typical surgical oncology patient at our center is a patient with pancreatic cancer for whom a Whipple procedure is recommended. Although blood loss in this setting is highly variable, we have previously reported the median intraoperative blood loss for this procedure to be 470 mL, or about 10% of total blood volume for the average-sized patient.[13] Thus, the Hb concentration should decrease by about 10% or from approximately 13 to 11.5 g/dL. However, we usually see about twice this amount of decrease over the entire hospital stay for several reasons. It has been said that all bleeding stops, but it does not exactly stop when the patient leaves the operating room. Patients may continue to bleed (albeit slowly) after surgery and the amount is difficult to measure because it does not all come out through the surgical drains. Three other issues come into play as well. There is hemodilution from intravenous (IV) fluids causing a postoperative downward Hb drift,[14] ongoing phlebotomy blood losses,[15] and impaired erythropoiesis in the setting of surgical stress and inflammation.[16] Because people destroy and create about 1% of their red blood cells every day, impaired erythropoiesis becomes problematic. For these 4 reasons, the Hb concentration generally trends downward while surgical patients are in the hospital.[17]

One tool the authors use to estimate potential blood loss of a given surgery is our maximum surgical blood order schedule.[13] This schedule is an institution-specific, data-driven list of all the different types of surgery along with the recommended preoperative blood orders. The cases are divided into 3 groups according to the potential for blood loss and likelihood of transfusion, which include no sample needed (low blood loss), type and screen (medium blood loss), and type and crossmatch (high blood loss). For example, the thyroidectomy is designated as low blood loss, whereas a Whipple or liver resection is considered high blood loss, and these categories are used to choose an appropriate preoperative Hb target.

The authors recently described their methods and treatment algorithms for managing preoperative anemia in bloodless surgery patients (**Fig. 3**).[18] Many patients with cancer, whether it be colorectal, pancreatic, or hepatobiliary, are malnourished in general, or perhaps losing blood slowly through the gastrointestinal tract, making them iron deficient. Some patients have undergone preoperative neoadjuvant myelosuppressive chemotherapy and are further predisposed to anemia. For the higher blood loss cases, an iron panel can be included automatically with their preoperative testing so they do not have to return for a second blood draw if their Hb level is low. Although

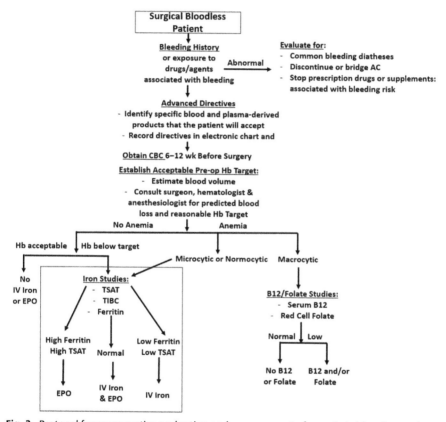

Fig. 3. Protocol for preoperative evaluation and management of anemia in bloodless patients. Laboratory studies, including a complete blood count with red blood cell indices and iron studies, are obtained for all patients as early as possible before a planned surgery. Patients with isolated iron deficiency are treated with parenteral iron alone, and those with anemia of chronic inflammation are treated with erythropoietin and parenteral iron, although attempts are made to avoid erythropoietin in patients with cancer who are having surgery with curative intent; they receive iron only. Patients with cancer who are unable to undergo surgery without higher Hb levels are offered therapy with erythropoietin (EPO) because they prefer to accept the potential risks of EPO therapy rather than the risks of not undergoing surgery. AC, anticoagulation; CBC, complete blood count; IV, intravenous; Pre-op, preoperative; TIBC, total iron binding capacity; TSAT, percentage of transferrin saturation. (*Adapted from* Chaturvedi S, Koo M, Dackiw L, et al. Preoperative treatment of anemia and outcomes in surgical Jehovah's Witness patients. Am J Hematol 2019;94(2):E56; with permission.)

microcytosis on the complete blood count can indicate chronic iron deficiency, the single best test to evaluate iron stores is a ferritin level. A ferritin level less than 20 ng/mL is low, and most anemic patients with low ferritin improve with IV iron replacement.[19] Importantly, ferritin is an acute phase reactant and levels are often increased in patients with underlying cancer and/or other chronic diseases. For these patients, the authors evaluate the transferrin saturation as a surrogate for available iron for erythropoiesis. Thus, patients with an increased ferritin levels (100–200 ng/mL) can have low transferrin saturations (<20%) associated with a functional iron deficiency and respond to iron therapy. For mildly anemic or mildly iron-deficient patients undergoing lower blood loss procedures, oral iron replacement may be sufficient, but several weeks may be required to increase the Hb level. Usually this is prescribed as 65 mg of elemental iron per dose (in the form of 325 mg of iron sulfate) to be taken with vitamin C or orange juice, which increases absorption.[18] Given the low percentage absorption, along with the moderate incidence of gastrointestinal intolerance (bloating, constipation, cramping), as well as some urgency to prepare patients before surgery, many centers treat with IV iron. There are too many different IV iron preparations to review here, but in general the highest single dose can be given with the newer low-molecular-weight iron dextran (InFed; Allergan, Madison, NJ). This preparation is most convenient for preoperative outpatient treatment because a single 1000-mg dose is often enough to fully replete a patient's iron stores.[20] Recently approved for iron deficiency is ferumoxytol (Feraheme; AMAG Pharmaceuticals, Lexington, MA), which can be given as a 510-mg dose. These preparations are typically used in the preoperative setting because the maximum single dose of iron sucrose (Venofer, American Regent, Shirley, NY) is only 200 to 300 mg, thus requiring repeated outpatient visits to achieve iron repletion. The authors use IV iron sucrose primarily for daily treatment of inpatients with iron deficiency. A rule of thumb is that, for each unit of blood that is lost in surgical patients (500 mL), 250 mg of iron replacement should be given to maintain iron stores.[21] Although IV iron preparations carry US Food and Drug Administration (FDA) warnings about hypersensitivity or anaphylactic-type reactions, these were much more common with high-molecular-weight iron dextran compounds,[20] which have been taken off the market.

For those patients with severe anemia or those with a very high target Hb level because of higher expected blood loss, erythropoiesis-stimulating agents (ESAs) may be considered. Erythropoietin and darbepoetin are the two primary medications used for bloodless patients. The primary concern with using ESAs is the FDA warning released in 2007 (http://www.janssenlabels.com/package-insert/product-mono graph/prescribing-information/PROCRIT-pi.pdf) that includes promotion of tumor growth, as well as thrombotic events.[22] Given this black box FDA warning, the risks and benefits of ESA treatment should be assessed on an individual case-by-case basis. The authors often reserve ESAs for surgical oncology patients who are being treated without curative intent; for example, those with metastatic disease.[9,10] Regarding the risk of thrombotic events, it is recommended that prophylactic anticoagulation be considered when ESAs are given as long as there is no significant active bleeding. When ESAs are given to oncology patients, we choose the lowest effective dose, which is often combined with IV iron, to increase effectiveness, because functional iron deficiency has been described in patients with cancer-associated anemia.[23–25] With aggressive iron or iron plus ESA therapy, typical iron-deficient patients increase their Hb levels about 1 to 1.5 g/dL each week.[18] Thus 3 to 4 weeks of therapy is usually adequate to treat mild to moderate preoperative anemia.

Dietary, herbal, or homeopathic supplements that may increase bleeding have been extensively reviewed,[26] and there are about 30 such compounds that may promote bleeding. With a cancer diagnosis, patients may be more likely to take these supplements seeking benefit, and it has been recommended to stop these for 2 to 3 weeks before surgery. Some commonly taken supplements that may promote bleeding, include bilberry, chamomile, dandelion root, dong quoi, garlic, ginger, ginseng, gingko, grape seed extract, horse chestnut, licorice, saw palmetto, oil of wintergreen, vitamin E, fish oil, chondroitin, and glucosamine.[27]

INTRAOPERATIVE ANESTHETIC MANAGEMENT

The primary goal of bloodless cancer surgery is keeping the blood in the patient. Simple methods, such as maintaining normothermia, are effective to reduce bleeding, because bleeding has been shown to increase at less than 35°C,[28,29] and has even been reported to increase at less than 36°C.[30] Controlled mild or moderate hypotension can also be helpful, especially for orthopedic or spine surgery, in which bone bleeding occurs. Such bleeding depends especially on blood pressure because bone cannot be cauterized, clamped, or sutured like other tissues.

More involved blood conservation methods can be initiated by the anesthesia team, such as ANH.[31] Although it is controversial whether this method is effective, the concept is physiologically plausible and is likely effective in certain cases. ANH is done by phlebotomy of autologous whole blood into citrate anticoagulant bags after anesthetic induction, followed by replacement of the patient's blood volume with crystalloid and/or colloid, thus intentionally decreasing the hematocrit during the blood loss portion of surgery. The patient therefore loses fewer red blood cells, and, after the bleeding is finished, the autologous whole blood is reinfused. The benefits are not only conservation of red blood cells but also that the fresh autologous whole blood is rich in clotting factors and platelets, making it superior to banked red cells or salvaged (cell saver) blood. The effectiveness of ANH requires 3 prerequisites:

1. A healthy starting Hb level
2. A high blood loss
3. The removal of large amounts of whole blood

Without all 3 of these, ANH is less safe and less effective in achieving the goal of blood conservation.

Another method for reducing blood loss and the likelihood of transfusion is the use of antifibrinolytics such as aminocaproic acid or tranexamic acid.[32] These lysine analogues have been around for more than 50 years, but only in the last 10 years have they been recognized as "game changers" resulting in reduced blood loss and transfusion requirements. Although they are most commonly used for orthopedic,[33] cardiac,[34] and trauma surgeries,[35] as well as for postpartum hemorrhage,[36] there is also potential benefit by reducing bleeding in liver or spine procedures, which are often performed for oncology patients. Studies comparing antifibrinolytics with placebo have shown an overall 30% reduction in bleeding and transfusion rates, and large randomized trials in trauma and postpartum hemorrhage have not shown an increase in thrombotic events.[35,36] Antifibrinolytics are relatively contraindicated in patients with active thrombosis and there is also increased risk of seizures with tranexamic acid at higher doses.[34,37]

INTRAOPERATIVE SURGICAL MANAGEMENT

There are several ways that surgeons can keep the blood in the patient, a primary goal of improving outcomes with bloodless surgery. The first method has been described as meticulous surgical technique. Although it could be argued that this is essential for all patients, it becomes evident that often blood loss is inversely proportional to how hard the surgeons try to reduce bleeding. For example, Whipple patients who are JWs may lose half as much blood as other Whipple patients. Whether it is tying off small bleeders, or more aggressive cauterization, or even letting more experienced providers do the cutting and suturing, something occurs that reduces bleeding.

Minimally invasive approaches, such as thoracoscopic, laparoscopic, and robotic surgery, have dramatically reduced bleeding. These approaches are now more commonly used in cancer surgery, especially for lung, prostate, and gynecologic procedures, but also more recently for colorectal, pancreatic, and hepatobiliary cancers. When first introduced, the operative time was substantially higher with these approaches, but robotic prostatectomies, for example, are now done in less than 2 to 3 hours and are associated with transfusion rates of less than 1%.[13] When open prostatectomy was the standard approach in the 1980s and 1990s, the transfusion rate was almost 100% and blood losses averaged close to 2 L.[38] Now even Whipple procedures and distal pancreatectomies are performed robotically with significantly lower blood losses. Hysterectomies are also routinely now done robotically with transfusion rates approaching zero. What at first seemed like a marketing tool, with claims of going home or back to work sooner, has now resulted in dramatically reduced blood loss and transfusion rates. The primary difference between open and robotic surgery may be the rates of blood loss and transfusion, because going home and back to work quickly is often not the primary concern of patients undergoing cancer surgery.

Not to be overlooked or underestimated are the topical hemostatic agents and the newer, more advanced versions of electrocautery. Topical hemostatics come in many varieties but usually comprise a gelatin matrix and a thrombin component.[39] Absorbable gelatin (Gelfoam, Pharmacia and Upjohn Co., Kalamazoo, MI) soaked in thrombin is commonly used and thrombin is now made with recombinant methods and not derived from human blood, making this acceptable even for JW patients who do not accept the minor fractions of blood. Premixed formulations of topical hemostatic agents, which include a predefined ratio of bovine-derived collagen and human thrombin, are now available in a syringe for easy application. However, clinicians should be extra careful to use a waste suction along with copious irrigation to avoid introducing topical hemostatic agents into the cell salvage reservoir (discussed later) because this can be associated with intravascular thrombosis.[40,41]

Newer cauteries, such as harmonic scalpels or saline irrigated bipolar cauteries, seal blood vessels rather than cutting or burning them, which results in reduced bleeding. These devices are routinely used for some head and neck cancer surgeries, as well as hepatic resections and some spine and orthopedic procedures. The authors have shown that using such specialized cautery results in a substantial reduction in blood loss and transfusion requirements (about 50%) with multilevel spine surgeries, which are often performed in oncology patients with spinal tumors or metastases.[42]

AUTOLOGOUS CELL SALVAGE

Blood salvage (often termed cell saver) has been around since the mid-1970s, when Haemonetics introduced the first device that washed shed blood using a conical centrifuge bowl. This device is designed to collect the blood via a suction catheter leading to a reservoir with a continuous flow of anticoagulant flowing down the suction tubing. The most common anticoagulant is heparin, although citrate can also be used. The blood is washed with saline to remove debris such as tissue or fat particles, and/or bone fragments. The centrifuge bowl also separates the red blood cells from the plasma and platelets, the latter of which are rinsed out into a waste bag during the washing and processing cycle lasting 10 to 15 minutes. What remains is a cell saver return product containing red blood cells and saline, with a typical hematocrit of 50% to 60%.

The absolute risk/benefit ratio for cell salvage has not been clearly determined for patients undergoing cancer surgery.[43,44] The primary concern is that reinfusing cancer cells into the systemic circulation could promote metastasis. This theoretic concern stems from a single case report in 1975 of a patient who died of metastatic lung cancer 4 weeks after pneumonectomy surgery.[45] Recently, case series have reported on the safety of using cell salvage for prostate cancer surgery; however, this particular cancer is most often contained within the prostate capsule at the time of diagnosis and surgery. Proponents of cell salvage for cancer surgery cite studies showing that circulating cancer cells are already present in the bloodstream at the time of surgery,[46,47] claiming that reinfusion of such cells does not increase risk.

Although this is a controversial area, the safety of salvaged blood in cancer surgery may be improved using a leukoreduction filter to reduce cancer cell exposure,[43,48] or by gamma irradiation of the processed salvaged blood before transfusing it back to the patient.[49] Several clinical studies support the safety of cell salvage in cancer surgery. In radical hysterectomy and gynecologic malignancy, survival and cancer recurrence rates were unchanged and no viable tumor cells were found when a leukoreduction filter was used.[50] Cell salvage also seems to be safe in urologic surgery for prostate and bladder cancer because disease recurrence and survival rates, as well as biochemical recurrence, were not increased.[51–53] In spine tumor surgery, cell salvage combined with leukoreduction filters resulted in no viable malignant cells in the finished salvaged product.[54] Given that allogeneic transfusion has been associated with increased cancer recurrence through transfusion-related immune modulation,[55] salvaged blood may be preferable, but prospective studies are needed to answer this question.

PHLEBOTOMY BLOOD LOSS

As previously stated, but worth restating, the primary goal is keeping the blood in the patient. A prime example is reducing blood loss caused by phlebotomy for laboratory testing. It is well known that phlebotomy blood losses during hospitalization can be substantial.[15] Standing daily laboratory orders are particularly problematic, as is the use of the larger phlebotomy tubes. The authors have shown that in our adult intensive care units (ICUs) at Johns Hopkins, typical patients lose about 60 mL/d because of laboratory testing (**Fig. 4**),[12] including the blood that is sent to the laboratory along with wasted blood that is discarded when clearing saline from the arterial or central line tubing. Using smaller phlebotomy tubes along with less frequent laboratory draws are two solutions to the problem.[56] Phlebotomy tubes come in 3 general sizes, adult, pediatric, and neonatal, which range from 6 to 10 mL, 2 to 5 mL, and 0.5 mL, respectively. Neonatal tubes are unpopular with phlebotomists and laboratories because they do not run through standard automated laboratory analyzers and must be run manually. They also lack a rubber stopper on top and must be uncapped to squirt the blood in, thus risking a splash exposure. For these reasons, the authors reserve the neonatal tubes for JW patients in the ICUs, and have generally switched to pediatric tubes (medium-sized tubes) throughout our hospital.

HEMOGLOBIN-BASED OXYGEN CARRIERS

One additional measure to consider is the availability and potential use of Hb-based oxygen carriers (HBOCs).[57] These compounds at times are referred to as blood

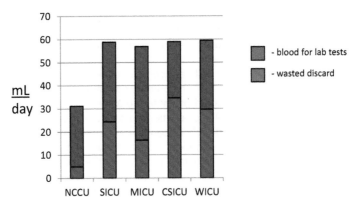

Fig. 4. Volume of blood removed from a patient in a 24-hour period in 5 different intensive care units at the Johns Hopkins Hospital. The blue portion is the wasted discard for clearing indwelling catheters of saline to provide an undiluted sample. The red portion is the volume of blood sent to the laboratory for the ordered tests. Slightly more than 1% of total blood volume is removed each day from a typical adult-sized patient, which is the same amount of red blood cells destroyed and replaced each day by normal erythropoiesis. In 1 ICU (the NCCU), an in-line blood-return device is routinely used, which reduces the blood volume lost to wasted discard. CSICU, Cardiac surgery intensive care unit; MICU, Medical intensive care unit; NCCU, Neurocritical care unit; SICU, Surgical intensive care unit; WICU, Weinberg intensive care unit. (*Data from* Frank SM, Scott AV, Resar LMS. Bloodless medicine and surgery: Top 10 things to consider. Anesthesia Experts. Available at: http://anesthesiaexperts. com/uncategorized/bloodless-medicine-surgery-top-10/. Accessed Jan 12 2019.)

substitutes or artificial blood. About 15 years ago, these were tested in multiple clinical trials but were not approved by the FDA because of concern about safety compared with conventional banked blood transfusions.[58] The HBOC products are polymerized or cross-linked bovine or human Hb molecules, with a half-life of about 24 hours. The primary concern in previous studies was unwanted vasoconstriction caused by nitric oxide scavenging, and the potential for vital organ ischemia. Recently, HBOC products have made a resurgence in a second round of submissions to the FDA, because it was realized that the control comparison group should have been no transfusion instead of banked blood, because the HBOC compounds are being targeted for those patients in whom transfusion is not an option because of red cell antibodies or unwillingness to accept allogeneic blood.

Although acceptance of HBOCs by JW patients is considered a personal choice, in our experience many have considered these to be a minor fraction and accept them. The only way to obtain HBOCs at this time is through single patient emergency compassionate use protocols, requiring FDA and institutional review board approval each time the HBOC is needed. It is hoped that, in the near future, HBOCs will be made available for acute life-threatening anemia when blood is not an option.

SUMMARY

Patients presenting for cancer surgery present a challenge when transfusion is not an option either for religious or personal reasons, or because of alloantibodies. Such bloodless surgery patients can be managed successfully using the methods described here and the outcomes can be equal or even superior to those of patients who accept transfusions. Through a multidisciplinary patient-centered approach, designed around managing preoperative anemia, keeping the blood in the patient, and sometimes tolerating lower Hb levels than usual, these patients can receive high-quality care. Many of the methods described for bloodless oncology patients can be applied to all patients, even when they accept transfusion, to reduce overall blood use along with its associated risks and costs, and by doing so clinicians improve the value of the health care they deliver.

ACKNOWLEDGMENTS

This work was partially funded by a grant from the New York Community Trust (NY, NY).

REFERENCES

1. Gross JB. Estimating allowable blood loss: corrected for dilution. Anesthesiology 1983;58:277–80.
2. Ott DA, Cooley DA. Cardiovascular surgery in Jehovah's Witnesses. Report of 542 operations without blood transfusion. JAMA 1977;238:1256–8.
3. Carson JL, Guyatt G, Heddle NM, et al. Clinical practice guidelines from the AABB: red blood cell transfusion thresholds and storage. JAMA 2016;316:2025–35.
4. Carson JL, Triulzi DJ, Ness PM. Indications for and adverse effects of red-cell transfusion. N Engl J Med 2017;377:1261–72.
5. Sadana D, Pratzer A, Scher LJ, et al. Promoting high-value practice by reducing unnecessary transfusions with a patient blood management program. JAMA Intern Med 2018;178:116–22.
6. Frank SM, Wick EC, Dezern AE, et al. Risk-adjusted clinical outcomes in patients enrolled in a bloodless program. Transfusion 2014;54:2668–77.
7. Pattakos G, Koch CG, Brizzio ME, et al. Outcome of patients who refuse transfusion after cardiac surgery: a natural experiment with severe blood conservation. Arch Intern Med 2012;172:1154–60.
8. Frank SM, Thakkar RN, Podlasek SJ, et al. Implementing a health system-wide patient blood management program with a clinical community approach. Anesthesiology 2017;127:754–64.
9. Resar LM, Frank SM. Bloodless medicine: what to do when you can't transfuse. Hematology Am Soc Hematol Educ Program 2014;2014:553–8.
10. Resar LM, Wick EC, Almasri TN, et al. Bloodless medicine: current strategies and emerging treatment paradigms. Transfusion 2016;56:2637–47.
11. Blood fractions and surgical procedures. Available at: https://wol.jw.org/en/wol/d/r1/lp-e/1102008086. Accessed January, 12, 2019.
12. Frank SM, Scott AV, Resar LM. Bloodless medicine and surgery: top 10 things to consider. Anesthesiology News 2016. Available at: http://anesthesiaexperts.com/uncategorized/bloodless-medicine-surgery-top-10/. Accessed January, 12, 2019.
13. Frank SM, Rothschild JA, Masear CG, et al. Optimizing preoperative blood ordering with data acquired from an anesthesia information management system. Anesthesiology 2013;118:1286–97.
14. Grant MC, Whitman GJ, Savage WJ, et al. Clinical predictors of postoperative hemoglobin drift. Transfusion 2014;54:1460–8.
15. Koch CG, Reineks EZ, Tang AS, et al. Contemporary bloodletting in cardiac surgical care. Ann Thorac Surg 2015;99:779–84.
16. Corwin HL. Anemia in the critically ill: the role of erythropoietin. Semin Hematol 2001;38:24–32.

17. Koch CG, Li L, Sun Z, et al. From bad to worse: anemia on admission and hospital-acquired anemia. J Patient Saf 2017;13:211–6.
18. Chaturvedi S, Koo M, Dackiw L, et al. Preoperative treatment of anemia and outcomes in surgical Jehovah's Witness patients. Am J Hematol 2019;94:E55–8.
19. Goodnough LT, Shander A. Patient blood management. Anesthesiology 2012; 116:1367–76.
20. Auerbach M, Pappadakis JA, Bahrain H, et al. Safety and efficacy of rapidly administered (one hour) one gram of low molecular weight iron dextran (INFeD) for the treatment of iron deficient anemia. Am J Hematol 2011;86:860–2.
21. Auerbach M. Intravenous iron in the perioperative setting. Am J Hematol 2014; 89:933.
22. Steinbrook R. Erythropoietin, the FDA, and oncology. N Engl J Med 2007;356: 2448–51.
23. Rodgers GM 3rd, Becker PS, Blinder M, et al. Cancer- and chemotherapy-induced anemia. J Natl Compr Canc Netw 2012;10:628–53.
24. Gilreath JA, Stenehjem DD, Rodgers GM. Diagnosis and treatment of cancer-related anemia. Am J Hematol 2014;89:203–12.
25. Henry DH, Dahl NV, Auerbach M, et al. Intravenous ferric gluconate significantly improves response to epoetin alfa versus oral iron or no iron in anemic patients with cancer receiving chemotherapy. Oncologist 2007;12:231–42.
26. Wong WW, Gabriel A, Maxwell GP, et al. Bleeding risks of herbal, homeopathic, and dietary supplements: a hidden nightmare for plastic surgeons? Aesthet Surg J 2012;32:332–46.
27. American Society of Anesthesiologists Task Force on Perioperative Blood Management. Practice guidelines for perioperative blood management: an updated report by the American Society of Anesthesiologists Task Force on Perioperative Blood Management*. Anesthesiology 2015;122:241–75.
28. Michelson AD, MacGregor H, Barnard MR, et al. Reversible inhibition of human platelet activation by hypothermia in vivo and in vitro. Thromb Haemost 1994; 71:633–40.
29. Rohrer MJ, Natale AM. Effect of hypothermia on the coagulation cascade. Crit Care Med 1992;20:1402–5.
30. Rajagopalan S, Mascha E, Na J, et al. The effects of mild perioperative hypothermia on blood loss and transfusion requirement. Anesthesiology 2008;108:71–7.
31. Grant MC, Resar LM, Frank SM. The efficacy and utility of acute normovolemic hemodilution. Anesth Analg 2015;121:1412–4.
32. Goobie SM, Frank SM. Tranexamic acid: what is known and unknown, and where do we go from here? Anesthesiology 2017;127:405–7.
33. Zufferey PJ, Miquet M, Quenet S, et al. Tranexamic acid in hip fracture surgery: a randomized controlled trial. Br J Anaesth 2010;104:23–30.
34. Myles PS, Smith JA, Forbes A, et al. Tranexamic acid in patients undergoing coronary-artery surgery. N Engl J Med 2017;376:136–48.
35. Roberts I, Shakur H, Afolabi A, et al. The importance of early treatment with tranexamic acid in bleeding trauma patients: an exploratory analysis of the CRASH-2 randomised controlled trial. Lancet 2011;377:1096–101, 1101.e1-2.
36. Collaborators WT. Effect of early tranexamic acid administration on mortality, hysterectomy, and other morbidities in women with post-partum haemorrhage (WOMAN): an international, randomised, double-blind, placebo-controlled trial. Lancet 2017;389:2105–16.
37. Goobie SM. Tranexamic acid: still far to go. Br J Anaesth 2017;118:293–5.

38. Shir Y, Raja SN, Frank SM, et al. Intraoperative blood loss during radical retropubic prostatectomy: epidural versus general anesthesia. Urology 1995;45:993–9.
39. Spotnitz WD, Burks S. Hemostats, sealants, and adhesives III: a new update as well as cost and regulatory considerations for components of the surgical toolbox. Transfusion 2012;52:2243–55.
40. Esper SA, Waters JH. Intra-operative cell salvage: a fresh look at the indications and contraindications. Blood Transfus 2011;9:139–47.
41. Sikorski RA, Rizkalla NA, Yang WW, et al. Autologous blood salvage in the era of patient blood management. Vox Sang 2017;112:499–510.
42. Frank SM, Wasey JO, Dwyer IM, et al. Radiofrequency bipolar hemostatic sealer reduces blood loss, transfusion requirements, and cost for patients undergoing multilevel spinal fusion surgery: a case control study. J Orthop Surg Res 2014; 9:50.
43. Waters JH, Donnenberg AD. Blood salvage and cancer surgery: should we do it? Transfusion 2009;49:2016–8.
44. Waters JH, Yazer M, Chen YF, et al. Blood salvage and cancer surgery: a meta-analysis of available studies. Transfusion 2012;52:2167–73.
45. Yaw PB, Sentany M, Link WJ, et al. Tumor cells carried through autotransfusion. Contraindication to intraoperative blood recovery? JAMA 1975;231:490–1.
46. Salsbury AJ. The significance of the circulating cancer cell. Cancer Treat Rev 1975;2:55–72.
47. Cole WH. The mechanisms of spread of cancer. Surg Gynecol Obstet 1973;137: 853–71.
48. Catling S, Williams S, Freites O, et al. Use of a leucocyte filter to remove tumour cells from intra-operative cell salvage blood. Anaesthesia 2008;63:1332–8.
49. Beck-Schimmer B, Romero B, Booy C, et al. Release of inflammatory mediators in irradiated cell salvage blood and their biological consequences in human beings following transfusion. Eur J Anaesthesiol 2004;21:46–52.
50. Connor JP, Morris PC, Alagoz T, et al. Intraoperative autologous blood collection and autotransfusion in the surgical management of early cancers of the uterine cervix. Obstet Gynecol 1995;86:373–8.
51. Nieder AM, Manoharan M, Yang Y, et al. Intraoperative cell salvage during radical cystectomy does not affect long-term survival. Urology 2007;69:881–4.
52. Stoffel JT, Topjian L, Libertino JA. Analysis of peripheral blood for prostate cells after autologous transfusion given during radical prostatectomy. BJU Int 2005; 96:313–5.
53. Davis M, Sofer M, Gomez-Marin O, et al. The use of cell salvage during radical retropubic prostatectomy: does it influence cancer recurrence? BJU Int 2003; 91:474–6.
54. Kumar N, Ahmed Q, Lee VK, et al. Can there be a place for intraoperative salvaged blood in spine tumor surgery? Ann Surg Oncol 2014;21:2436–43.
55. Amato A, Pescatori M. Perioperative blood transfusions for the recurrence of colorectal cancer. Cochrane Database Syst Rev 2006;(1):CD005033.
56. Koch CG, Li L, Sun Z, et al. Hospital-acquired anemia: prevalence, outcomes, and healthcare implications. J Hosp Med 2013;8:506–12.
57. Weiskopf RB. Hemoglobin-based oxygen carriers: compassionate use and compassionate clinical trials. Anesth Analg 2010;110:659–62.
58. Natanson C, Kern SJ, Lurie P, et al. Cell-free hemoglobin-based blood substitutes and risk of myocardial infarction and death: a meta-analysis. JAMA 2008;299: 2304–12.

Therapeutic Utility of Cold-Stored Platelets or Cold-Stored Whole Blood for the Bleeding Hematology-Oncology Patient

Thomas G. Scorer, MBBS, FRCPath[a,b],*,
Kristin M. Reddoch-Cardenas, PhD[c], Kimberly A. Thomas, PhD[d],
Andrew P. Cap, MD, PhD[c], Philip C. Spinella, MD, FCCM[d]

KEYWORDS

- Cold-stored platelets • Platelet transfusion • Platelet storage • Bleeding
- Thrombocytopenia • Oncology

KEY POINTS

- The management of bleeding caused by thrombocytopenia is a significant problem for hematology-oncology patients.
- The current standard of care, room temperature stored platelets, is suboptimal because of the platelet storage lesion, risk of bacterial contamination, and short shelf-life.
- When compared with the standard of care, cold stored platelets have displayed enhanced hemostatic properties, including aggregation, clot strength, clot retraction, and adhesion under flow.

Continued

Disclosure Statement: T.G. Scorer, K.M. Reddoch-Cardenas, K.A. Thomas, and A.P. Cap have no conflicts of interest to disclose. P.C. Spinella serves as consultant for Cerus and Hemanext. P.C. Spinella has received research support from Terumo BCT.
Disclaimers: The opinions or assertions expressed herein are the private views of the authors and are not to be construed as official or as reflecting the views of the US Department of the Army, the US Department of Defense, the Ministry of Defence, the National Institute for Health Research, or the Department of Health.
[a] School of Cellular and Molecular Medicine, University of Bristol, Bristol Royal Infirmary, Research Floor 7, Queens Building, Bristol, BS2 8HW, UK; [b] Centre of Defence Pathology, Royal Centre for Defence Medicine, Birmingham, UK; [c] Coagulation and Blood Research, U.S. Army Institute of Surgical Research, 3698 Chambers Pass, BLDG 3610, JBSA-Fort Sam Houston, San Antonio, TX 78234, USA; [d] Department of Pediatrics, Division of Pediatric Critical Care Medicine, Washington University School of Medicine, 660 South Euclid Avenue, St. Louis, MO 63110, USA
* Corresponding author. Bristol Royal Infirmary, Research Floor 7, Queens Building, Bristol, BS2 8HW, UK.
E-mail address: tom.scorer@bristol.ac.uk

Hematol Oncol Clin N Am 33 (2019) 873–885
https://doi.org/10.1016/j.hoc.2019.05.012
0889-8588/19/© 2019 Elsevier Inc. All rights reserved.

Continued

- Additional benefits of cold stored platelets include lower transfusion-transmissible infections, reduced thrombotic risk, a preferable immunologic profile, and longer shelf-life.
- Studies should be performed to compare the efficacy of cold stored platelets and the standard of care at managing and preventing bleeding in hematology-oncology patients.

INTRODUCTION

Platelets are critical for clot formation and preventing uncontrolled bleeding. Produced in the bone marrow, platelets circulate in the bloodstream for 8 to 10 days and are constantly replenished to replace those that are removed from the circulation. Thrombocytopenia can occur because of either hereditary or acquired disorders. It can be caused by either reduced platelet production (eg, infiltration of the bone marrow and chemoradiotherapy) and/or increased consumption (eg, disseminated intravascular coagulation and severe bleeding). Thrombocytopenia is a common condition in hematology-oncology patients and increases the risk of life-threatening bleeding. In developed countries, patients with hematological malignancy comprise the majority of platelet transfusion episodes. It is currently estimated that 67% of all platelets are used to manage hematological malignancies, while the remaining platelets are predominantly used during cardiac surgery and in intensive care.[1–4]

Prophylactic transfusion for treatment of thrombocytopenia was first established in 1910 by W.W. Duke as a means to reduce bleeding risk, and by the 1960s platelet transfusion became standard practice for patients with a platelet count of less than 20×10^9/L.[5–7] Decades later, studies suggested that a restrictive platelet transfusion threshold of less than 10×10^9/L was safe for preventing bleeding in patients with acute myeloid leukemia.[8–10] As a result, more restrictive platelet transfusion guidelines are now in place in some countries.[11,12] These guidelines advocate a prophylactic platelet transfusion threshold of less than 10×10^9/L but only to those patients with reversible bone marrow failure receiving intensive chemotherapy or allogeneic bone marrow transplant.[3,9] In patients with asymptomatic, chronic bone marrow failure, including low-dose chemotherapy regimens and those undergoing uncomplicated autologous stem cell transplantation (ASCT), empirical prophylactic platelet transfusion is not recommended.[3,9] The standard of care, therefore, is transitioning from the majority of thrombocytopenic patients receiving prophylactic PLT transfusion toward a more restrictive approach with increasing numbers of patients only receiving PLT transfusions for active bleeding.

PREPARATION AND STORAGE OF PLATELET PRODUCTS FOR TRANSFUSION: THE CURRENT STANDARD OF CARE AND ITS DEFICIENCIES

Platelet concentrates (PCs) used for transfusion can be prepared from separation of whole blood (WB) by either the platelet-rich plasma (PRP) or buffy coat methods and pooled before administration; alternatively, platelets can be collected from single donors using apheresis. Superiority of 1 platelet product over the other in terms of hemostatic benefit, post-transfusion increments, and adverse events has not been shown. Often the choice of platelet product is made based on the cost of the collection, with pooled PCs being the least costly to produce. Geographic location also dictates choice of platelet collection method. For instance in the United States, platelet apheresis is dominant, and buffy coat-derived platelets are not licensed.[13] Lastly, platelet product manufacturing methods often depend on the condition being treated. For example, when histocompatible platelet transfusions are required, apheresis platelet collections become a necessity.[9]

Current storage guidelines for platelets date back to the late 1960s. In the first and most cited study, Murphy and Gardner infused small volumes of Chromium-51 labeled autologous platelets that had been stored for 8 or 18 hours at either room temperature (RT, 22°C) or cold temperature (4°C) into healthy donors and assessed the circulation times of the platelets.[14] This study determined that platelets stored in the cold had a reduced recovery and circulating half-life after infusion compared with those stored at RT, and further identified RT as the best storage temperature for maximizing platelet recovery and survival. Subsequent studies by others confirmed the reduced recovery and half-life of cold-stored platelets (CSPs) but also showed that CSPs displayed better hemostatic properties, both in vitro and in vivo, than room temperature platelets (RTPs).[15,16] Between the late 1970s and early 1980s, many blood transfusion laboratories maintained a dual platelet inventory, with platelets being stored at both RT and in the cold. However, because of the complexity and cost of maintaining dual inventories, and since the dominant clinical use of PLT transfusion at this time was empiric prophylactic transfusion to prevent spontaneous bleeding in thrombocytopenic patients, RTP storage became favored practice.

RTPs stored in gas-permeable bags with agitation have a maximum shelf life of approximately 3 to 7 days (3 days in Japan; 4 days in Germany; 5 days in Australia; and 7 days in Canada, Netherlands, the United Kingdom, and the United States [7 days in the United States if point-of-release bacterial testing is used; otherwise the shelf life is 5 days]).[17] PCs can be stored in either 100% plasma or with a portion of the plasma replaced by a platelet-additive solution (PAS), a technique known to help better preserve platelet shelf life and reduce transfusion-related reactions.[18] These restrictions in shelf life for RTPs are primarily because of an increased risk of bacterial contamination. Platelet products are the leading cause of blood product-transmitted bacterial infections; various studies report that an estimated 1 in 5000 PLT units are bacterially contaminated in the United States alone, with 1 in 100,000 platelet transfusions resulting in sepsis.[19–22] Extended storage of platelet units at RT allows for clinically significant proliferation of even the smallest bacterial inoculums.[21] Furthermore, WB-derived platelets are associated with a fivefold higher contamination rate than single-donor apheresis-derived platelets due to the increased number of venipunctures involved in the preparation of pooled platelet products.[21,22] Bacterial screening of all platelet units is thereby considered a requirement and incurs significant cost and logistical burdens. Further, bacterial screening requires quarantining. Despite enforcement of increased hemovigilance and screening, the risk for fatalities remains. Pathogen inactivation (PI) methods or pathogen reduction technologies (PRTs) can presumably alleviate some of the concerns of bacterial contamination at RT but have been shown to impair in vitro PLT function and also result in smaller count increments after transfusion in nonbleeding patients.[23–28] Interestingly, in clinical studies comparing PRT platelets to standard platelets, outcomes are similar between groups.[29]

The limited shelf life of platelets places a huge strain on inventory management for hospitals and blood centers and leads to wastage, predominantly because of outdating, but also (although to a much lesser extent) recall for positive bacterial screening.[19] In 2015, US blood centers reported that outdated platelet units totaled 213,000, accounting for over a quarter of all platelet units and amounting to health care costs totaling an estimated $1 billion annually.[30,31] Further perpetuating a strained platelet inventory is an increase in the number of platelet transfusions performed. Between

2007 and 2014, the number of platelet transfusions increased by 25% because of a combination of an aging population, increased incidence of hypoproliferative thrombocytopenia, intensity of chemotherapy treatment, and number of indications for transfusion.[32] Even in developed countries, many blood centers remain unable to provide RTPs for life-threatening conditions (eg, trauma resuscitation) because of the short shelf life and logistical constraints. Instead, PLT transfusion has become the preserve of a small number of well-resourced centers with easy access to blood processing centers.[33] This causes smaller centers to deliver suboptimal care because of the inability to keep platelets in inventory and not have them available when needed for patients with life-threatening hemorrhage.

Additionally, during RTP storage, platelets exhibit various biophysical and biochemical changes that are collectively referred to as the platelet storage lesion (PSL).[34] The PSL begins with collection of the platelet unit; each of the collection methods (ie, buffy-coat, apheresis, and PRP method) requires the use of different centrifugation steps to isolate platelets and have been shown to result in varying degrees of centrifugation-induced activation of the platelets.[35,36] For example, exposure of CD62P (P-Selectin), activation of GPIIb/IIIa receptor, and shedding of GPIb have all been shown to occur more frequently with the collection of PRP-derived platelets compared with apheresis platelets.[17,36] Apart from collection-induced activation, platelet activation and the effects of PSL are highly evident with increased storage duration at RT. Storage for 5 days at RT leads to the release of granular contents, enhanced exposure of phosphatidylserine (PS) and P-Selectin, accumulation of immunomodulatory mediators, increased metabolic breakdown, and decreased hemostatic function.[37–42] The PSL may also have clinical consequences. Inaba and colleagues[43] reported in a retrospective study that after adjusting for severity of illness, trauma patients transfused platelets at 5 days of storage had increased incidence of sepsis compared with patients transfused platelets at 3 days of storage.

EFFICACY OF ROOM-TEMPERATURE PLATELETS IN TREATING HEMATOLOGY-ONCOLOGY PATIENTS

Hemostatic efficacy of platelet products should be of utmost priority when transfusing to thrombocytopenic patients. Of the limited randomized controlled trials (RCTs) that exist, the results vary as to whether prophylactic platelet transfusions actually help prevent bleeding in most hematology-oncology patients.[44–46] In Slichter and colleagues'[46] groundbreaking work, researchers assessed the effect of dose of prophylactically administered PLTs on bleeding in hypoproliferative thrombocytopenic patients (the PLADO study). It was hypothesized that administration of a high platelet dose would presumably offer superior hemostasis while a lower platelet dose, if effective, would conserve an already strained platelet supply. In actuality, platelet dose had no effect on the incidence of bleeding in this patient population; bleeding risk did not vary between a platelet count of 10×10^9-80×10^9/L, and risk of grade 2 bleeding was the same within 24 hours of transfusion as prior to transfusion.[46] A subsequent analysis of PLADO by Uhl and colleagues[47] showed that factors such as presence of coagulopathy (prolonged PT/aPTT) or hematocrit less than 25% or patient characteristics (allogeneic SCT [alloSCT] or induction chemotherapy vs autologous SCT) explained bleeding risk. Wandt and colleagues[12] (2012) and Stanworth and colleagues[11] (2013) showed independently that intensive chemotherapy and allogeneic stem cell transplant (alloSCT) patients derived benefit from prophylactic transfusion, whereas patients undergoing autologous SCT or other less-intensive regimens could be safely treated with therapeutic rather than prophylactic transfusions.

The value of platelet transfusion in other patient groups has also been reported with mixed outcomes. In a multicenter study by Curley and colleagues,[48] neonates with severe thrombocytopenia were transfused at a platelet-count threshold of 25×10^9/L (low threshold) or at 50×10^9/L (high-threshold) with incidence of bleeding documented. Of the 660 infants who underwent randomization, it was determined that those in the high-threshold group had a significantly higher rate of major bleeding or death than the low-threshold group.[48] In the PATCH study, an international, open-label RCT, patients presenting with intracranial hemorrhage (ICH) while on anti-PLT therapy were randomized to receive PLT transfusion (RTPs) or standard care.[49] The odds of death or dependence 3 months after ICH was higher in the platelet transfusion group.[49] This unexpected finding highlighted that RTP transfusion may cause harm in some patient groups. On the other hand, PLT transfusion in trauma patients with severe bleeding has been associated with improved outcomes.[50–52] In a secondary analysis in the PROPPR RCT, the group of patients receiving platelets had improved survival compared with patients who did not receive platelets.[53] Taken together, data from the aforementioned studies demonstrate that prophylactic platelet transfusions are necessary to prevent bleeding in some patients with very low counts ($<10 \times 10^9$/L) caused by intensive chemotherapy and in alloSCT; prophylaxis may be ineffective and possibly harmful in other populations, and use of RTP may be suboptimal for treatment of bleeding in patients without massive bleeding (ie, ICH as opposed to exsanguinating trauma patients).

REVISITING COLD STORED PLATELET AS AN ALTERNATIVE TO THE STANDARD OF CARE

Although use of RTPs has been the standard of care for several decades, interest in CSPs has now re-emerged because of increased use of platelet transfusions in actively bleeding patients, particularly following trauma, but also as a result of the disappointing findings related to RTP in nonmassively bleeding patients, as described previously (eg, ICH). There is now more evidence supporting the historical findings that CSPs have greater hemostatic properties. Numerous studies have reported that CSPs exhibit enhanced hemostatic properties over RTPs, including: aggregation, clot strength, clot retraction, and adhesion under flow.[37–41,54,55] Another feature of CSPs that has been widely reproduced is the upregulation of activation markers when compared with RTPs, both at baseline and following stimulation with agonists.[38,40,41,55–57] Despite this increase in activation markers, CSP show preserved response to endothelial inhibitors (ie, nitric oxide and prostacyclin) and thus presumably retain the ability to deliver hemostasis to sites of injury without causing thrombosis; this has been validated in a laser injury and intravital microscopy animal model in which no excessive thrombogenicity was observed with use of CSPs.[58,59] More recently, it has been reported that CSPs may confer an advantage over RTPs at reversing the effect of antiplatelet medications in vitro.[60,61] This adds to historical data reporting that bleeding times (BTs) in an RCT of healthy volunteers treated with aspirin were corrected to a greater extent following CSP transfusion compared with RTP transfusion.[16,62–64]

The increased hemostatic function of CSPs raises the possibility that CSPs could be more clinically effective than RTPs in the treatment of bleeding and that previous concerns about inferior pharmacokinetics are less relevant in the acute setting. Indeed, in the unwell hematology-oncology patient population, platelet survival is reduced with patients requiring regular RTP transfusion to maintain a platelet count and/or treat bleeding. Contemporary clinical evidence for CSPs in the hematology-oncology population is limited. Historically, few studies have reported the clinical effectiveness of

CSP versus RTP transfusion in thrombocytopenic patients, all published in the 1970s with conflicting conclusions. In the first of these, Becker and colleagues[16] reported transfusing 93 thrombocytopenic patients (80 with active bleeding and BT>15 s) a total of 107 units of platelets. The thrombocytopenic patients were reported to have a wide range of diagnoses (eg, acute leukemia, lymphoma, disseminated malignancy, and aplastic anemia), and patients were randomized to receive either CSP or RTP transfusions. Correction in BT and clinical bleeding assessments (clinician blinded to treatment) were utilized to assess clinical efficacy. In this study, CSPs corrected BTs in more patients than RTPs and improved clinical bleeding in more patients (84% vs 39%, respectively).[16] Slichter and Harker[64] assessed CSP and RTP transfusion by recording BTs in aplastic patients (diagnosis and number not reported) and demonstrated that CSP transfusion resulted in no measurable improvement in BTs or only transient improvements lasting less than 2.5 hours, whereas, RTP transfusion was reported to correct BT within 2.5 hours. Lastly, Filip and Aster[62] reported transfusion of CSPs and RTPs to 22 hypoproliferative thrombocytopenic patients (BTs>25 s with no evidence of alloimmunization). This study reported that there was no difference between RTPs and CSPs, 1 hour after transfusion.[62] An explanation for these differences could be related to the methods used to process the platelet concentrates, which varied significantly between these articles and utilized methods no longer employed in current platelet manufacture.

Outside of the hematology-oncology population, there is only a single contemporary pilot RCT of CSPs versus RTPs, which has recently been completed in cardiothoracic surgery patients. Although the study is due to report in full, provisional findings have reported reduced postoperative chest drain output with CSP use.[65] These promising preliminary findings prompted researchers to add a single-arm extension to assess the efficacy of 14 -day stored CSP versus a 7-day stored RTP product. Patients receiving CSP stored for 14 days had chest tube output comparable to those receiving RTP or CSP stored for 7 days, suggesting that extended cold storage of platelets may be possible.

As previously stated, CSPs were deemed unfavorable for use in both therapeutic and prophylactic settings for decades based on the short circulation time and more rapid clearance from the bloodstream, a process that involves platelet GPIbα.[31,66–71] Chilling of platelets leads to shedding of GPIbα from the platelet surface and also causes glycan modification of the receptor, including desialylation.[41,68–70,72,73] Desialylation results in clustering of GPIbα into lipid rafts that are targeted for clearance by liver macrophages or hepatocyte Ashwell-Morell receptors.[71,74,75] Although often perceived as unfavorable, the reduced circulation time of CSPs may confer an additional advantage over RTPs. Rapid clearance of CSPs from the circulation following a bleeding episode could reduce the risk of thrombosis following resuscitation. Hematology-oncology patients are often prothrombotic because of the inflammatory nature of malignant disease, anticancer therapies, immobilization, and the presence of central venous catheters. The occurrence of thrombosis increases morbidity and mortality and complicates the optimum delivery of anticancer therapy. Utilization of CSPs in this scenario would offer the best of both worlds: fast-acting management of bleeding and quick clearance of nonparticipating platelets that could reduce prothrombotic complications following a bleeding episode.

COLD STORED WHOLE BLOOD

When discussing PCs it is of value to also consider the transfusion of WB. WB can be transfused as warm fresh whole blood (FWB) in deployed military settings or following cold storage (CSWB). There is minimal evidence of WB usage in the hematology-oncology population. Historically, and prior to component therapy, WB was been shown to benefit patients compared with no transfusion therapy.[5] WB has also been reported to reduce bleeding compared with transfusion of blood components in a 1:1:1 unit ratio in an RCT of pediatric cardiac surgery patients.[76] If WB is stored in the cold, the PLTs exhibit similar characteristics to those in CSP. It has been demonstrated that the PLTs within CSWB contribute to clot formation to the same extent as those in FWB in trauma and hemorrhagic shock models.[59] The platelets within CSWB remain functional, and the hemostatic properties of CSWB are not compromised and likely superior to conventional component therapy.[77–80] Hematology-oncology patients often do not require all of the components of WB; however in the bleeding, pancytopenic patient, WB may be the optimum resuscitation fluid, because it minimizes donor exposure and reduces the risk of alloimmunization.

INFLAMMATORY AND IMMUNE EFFECTS OF COLD STORAGE

Although generally well-tolerated, PLT transfusions cause the most transfusion reactions of all blood products.[81] Typical adverse events that can occur from PLT transfusions include everything from fever and minor allergic reactions to much more serious events like transfusion-associated sepsis and transfusion-related acute lung injury (TRALI).[82] PCs consist of platelets, plasma, microparticles, and sometimes leukocytes if the unit has not been leukoreduced. Over the course of storage, platelets secrete soluble mediators such as soluble CD40L (sCD40L), which can accumulate in the PC supernatant. High sCD40L levels have been known to have a direct association with TRALI development and can induce febrile nonhemolytic reactions through activation of cyclooxygenase-2.[83,84] CSPs have been shown to have less accumulation of sCD40L than RTPs after 5 days of storage and are presumably less inflammatory.[41] Other common soluble inflammatory mediators that are released into the plasma supernatant during extended storage at RT include soluble thromboxane, P-Selectin (sP-selectin), platelet-derived growth factor (PDGF), vascular endothelial growth factor (VEGF), platelet factor 4 (PF4), and various cytokines (eg, interleukin [IL]-6 and IL-1β).[17,41,85] Increased soluble mediator release may be detrimental for hematologic malignancy patients receiving transfusions, as an increase in growth factors may actually stimulate tumor growth and counteract growth factor-targeted therapies.[85]

Research into the immunomodulatory state of CSP is currently lacking. Platelets play many roles in modulating leukocyte function, both indirectly through soluble mediators, as well as directly through receptor-mediated cell:cell interactions.[86,87] Cold storage of platelets increases surface expression of CD62P and CD40L which mediate platelet-leukocyte aggregates (PLAs)[88] formation through binding of cognate ligands, PSGL-1 and CD40, respectively.[89–91] PLA engagement causes intracellular signaling, which can result in NFκB activation and inflammatory cytokine production.[92,93] Moreover, PLAs are considered prothrombotic and proinflammatory.[88] Although work with CSWB has shown increased PLAs in vitro[94] and in vivo,[95] there is no literature examining whether CSPs result in increased PLA in vivo in healthy individuals, let alone patients with hematological malignancies. As PLAs can be prothrombotic and proinflammatory, the actual occurrence of this phenomenon in the context of CSP transfusion should be evaluated further.

As cold storage of platelets leads to increased PS expression[41,96] and more rapid clearance in vivo than their RT-stored counterparts,[14–16] it is important to understand the immune response during PS-mediated apoptotic cell clearance. Importantly, apoptotic clearance mechanisms reliant on PS recognition promote a strong anti-inflammatory response.[97] Specifically, engagement of myeloid-expressed scavenger receptors by PS results in intracellular signaling cascades that suppress TNF-α and IL-1β production and stimulate IL-10 production.[98,99] The increased PS expression by CSP and subsequent clearance-induced anti-inflammatory cascade thereby presents an opposite inflammatory phenomenon compared with that of PLA. Moreover, the pleiotropic effects of IL-10 in cancer[100] would further confound the potential immunologic effects of CSP in cancer patients receiving PLT transfusions. Therefore, the true nature of the immunomodulatory effect of PS-expressing CSPs remains to be defined.

Lastly, a study from Herzig, and colleagues[101] suggests that CSPs are not proinflammatory in a mixed lymphocyte reaction model (MLR). In this study, labeled peripheral blood mononuclear cells (PBMCs) were incubated with diluted apheresis platelets (in either 100% plasma or 65% PAS/35% plasma) stored at both RT and in the cold, and PBMC proliferation was determined after 96 hours. The addition of CSPs inhibited PBMC proliferation, suggesting a transfusion-related immunomodulation (TRIM) event. These potentially diametrically opposed effects of CSPs on immune function further suggest the need for mechanistic study to determine the true immunomodulatory potential of CSP in patients with hematological malignancies.

SUMMARY

As has been outlined in this article, RTP, the current standard of care in treatment of thrombocytopenic hematology-oncology patients is oftentimes unsuccessful and possibly even detrimental for the prevention or management of bleeding. Moving away from a predominantly prophylactic approach to platelet transfusion toward a more therapeutic strategy by use of a platelet product with superior hemostatic function should be evaluated in the hematology-oncology patient population. Use of CSPs in these patients would potentially offer a superior treatment to control active bleeding and confer a lower risk of transfusion-transmissible infections, reduced thrombotic risk, and a preferable immunologic profile. Furthermore, the logistical advantages of a longer shelf-life and simplified storage conditions would save money and improve outcomes for many patients who currently do not have access to any platelet transfusion therapy. Studies should be performed in hematology-oncology patients to compare CSPs versus RTPs in prophylactic and therapeutic treatment scenarios.

ACKNOWLEDGMENTS

T.G. Scorer was supported by the NIHR Biomedical Research Centre at University Hospitals Bristol NHS Foundation Trust and the University of Bristol.

REFERENCES

1. Cameron B, Rock G, Olberg B, et al. Evaluation of platelet transfusion triggers in a tertiary-care hospital. Transfusion 2007;47(2):206–11.
2. Charlton A, Wallis J, Robertson J, et al. Where did platelets go in 2012? A survey of platelet transfusion practice in the North of England. Transfus Med 2014; 24(4):213–8.
3. Estcourt LJ, Birchall J, Allard S, et al. Guidelines for the use of platelet transfusions. Br J Haematol 2017;176(3):365–94.
4. Greeno E, McCullough J, Weisdorf D. Platelet utilization and the transfusion trigger: a prospective analysis. Transfusion 2007;47(2):201–5.

5. Duke WW. The relation of blood platelets to hemorrhagic disease - description of a method for determining the bleeding time and coagulation time and report of three cases of hemorrhagic disease relieved by transfusion. J Am Med Assoc 1910;55:1185–92.

6. Gaydos LA, Mantel N, Freireich EJ. Quantitative relation between platelet count and hemorrhage in patients with acute leukemia. N Engl J Med 1962;266(18): 905–9.

7. Wandt H, Schafer-Eckart K, Greinacher A. Platelet transfusion in hematology, oncology and surgery. Dtsch Arztebl Int 2014;111(48):809–15.

8. Rebulla P, Finazzi G, Marangoni F, et al. The threshold for prophylactic platelet transfusions in adults with acute myeloid leukemia. N Engl J Med 1997;337(26): 1870–5.

9. Schiffer CA, Bohlke K, Delaney M, et al. Platelet transfusion for patients with cancer: American society of clinical oncology clinical practice guideline update. J Clin Oncol 2018;36(3):283–99.

10. Wandt H, Frank M, Ehninger G, et al. Safety and cost effectiveness of a 10 x 10(9)/L trigger for prophylactic platelet transfusions compared with the traditional 20 x 10(9)/L trigger: a prospective comparative trial in 105 patients with acute myeloid leukemia. Blood 1998;91(10):3601–6.

11. Stanworth SJ, Estcourt LJ, Powter G, et al. A no-prophylaxis platelet-transfusion strategy for hematologic cancers. N Engl J Med 2013;368(19):1771–80.

12. Wandt H, Schaefer-Eckart K, Wendelin K, et al. Therapeutic platelet transfusion versus routine prophylactic transfusion in patients with haematological malignancies: an open-label, multicentre, randomised study. Lancet 2012;380(9850): 1309–16.

13. Whitaker B, Rajbhandary S, Kleinman S, et al. Trends in United States blood collection and transfusion: results from the 2013 AABB blood collection, utilization, and patient blood management survey. Transfusion 2016;56(9):2173–83.

14. Murphy S, Gardner FH. Effect of storage temperature on maintenance of platelet viability–deleterious effect of refrigerated storage. N Engl J Med 1969;280(20): 1094–8.

15. Valeri CR. Hemostatic effectiveness of liquid-preserved and previously frozen human platelets. N Engl J Med 1974;290(7):353–8.

16. Becker GA, Tuccelli M, Kunicki T, et al. Studies of platelet concentrates stored at 22 C and 4 C. Transfusion 1973;13(2):61–8.

17. Ng MSY, Tung JP, Fraser JF. Platelet storage lesions: what more do we know now? Transfus Med Rev 2018. [Epub ahead of print].

18. Ringwald J, Zimmermann R, Eckstein R. The new generation of platelet additive solution for storage at 22 degrees C: Development and current experience. Transfus Med Rev 2006;20(2):158–64.

19. Brecher ME, Hay SN. Bacterial contamination of blood components. Clin Microbiol Rev 2005;18(1):195–204.

20. Horth RZ, Jones JM, Kim JJ, et al. Fatal sepsis associated with bacterial contamination of platelets - Utah and California, August 2017. MMWR Morb Mortal Wkly Rep 2018;67(25):718–22.

21. Canellini G, Waldvogel S, Anderegg K, et al. Bacterial contamination of platelet concentrates: perspectives for the future (vol 41, pg 301, 2010). Lab Med 2010; 41(7):439.

22. Ness P, Braine H, King K, et al. Single-donor platelets reduce the risk of septic platelet transfusion reactions. Transfusion 2001;41(7):857–61.

23. Osman A, Hitzler WE, Meyer CU, et al. Effects of pathogen reduction systems on platelet microRNAs, mRNAs, activation, and function. Platelets 2015;26(2):154–63.
24. Zeddies S, De Cuyper IM, van der Meer PF, et al. Pathogen reduction treatment using riboflavin and ultraviolet light impairs platelet reactivity toward specific agonists in vitro. Transfusion 2014;54(9):2292–300.
25. Cazenave JP, Follea G, Bardiaux L, et al. A randomized controlled clinical trial evaluating the performance and safety of platelets treated with MIRASOL pathogen reduction technology. Transfusion 2010;50(11):2362–75.
26. Kerkhoffs JLH, van Putten WLJ, Novotny VMJ, et al. Clinical effectiveness of leucoreduced, pooled donor platelet concentrates, stored in plasma or additive solution with and without pathogen reduction. Br J Haematol 2010;150(2):209–17.
27. Rebulla P, Vaglio S, Beccaria F, et al. Clinical effectiveness of platelets in additive solution treated with two commercial pathogen-reduction technologies. Transfusion 2017;57(5):1171–83.
28. van Rhenen D, Gulliksson H, Cazenave JP, et al. Transfusion of pooled buffy coat platelet components prepared with photochemical pathogen inactivation treatment: the euroSPRITE trial. Blood 2003;101(6):2426–33.
29. Nussbaumer W, Amato M, Schennach H, et al. Patient outcomes and amotosalen/UVA-treated platelet utilization in massively transfused patients. Vox Sang 2017;112(3):249–56.
30. Ellingson KD, Sapiano MRP, Haass KA, et al. Continued decline in blood collection and transfusion in the United States-2015. Transfusion 2017;57(Suppl 2):1588–98.
31. Hoffmeister KM, Felbinger TW, Falet H, et al. The clearance mechanism of chilled blood platelets. Cell 2003;112(1):87–97.
32. Estcourt LJ. Why has demand for platelet components increased? A review. Transfus Med 2014;24(5):260–8.
33. Cotton S, Hyam C. A survey of platelet inventory management in 228 hospitals. Transfus Med 2010;20(s1):26–54.
34. Devine DV, Serrano K. The platelet storage lesion. Clin Lab Med 2010;30(2):475–87.
35. Greening DW, Simpson RJ, Sparrow RL. Preparation of platelet concentrates for research and transfusion purposes. Methods Mol Biol 2017;1619:31–42.
36. Vassallo RR, Murphy S. A critical comparison of platelet preparation methods. Curr Opin Hematol 2006;13(5):323–30.
37. Bynum JA, Meledeo MA, Getz TM, et al. Bioenergetic profiling of platelet mitochondria during storage: 4 degrees C storage extends platelet mitochondrial function and viability. Transfusion 2016;56(Suppl 1):S76–84.
38. Montgomery RK, Reddoch KM, Evani SJ, et al. Enhanced shear-induced platelet aggregation due to low-temperature storage. Transfusion 2013;53(7):1520–30.
39. Nair PM, Pandya SG, Dallo SF, et al. Plasma factor XIII binding to cold-stored platelets results in increased fibrin crosslinking and clot strength. Arterioscl Throm Vas 2017;37:A147.
40. NasrEldin E. Effect of cold storage on platelets quality stored in a small containers: Implications for pediatric transfusion. Pediatr Hematol Oncol J 2017;2(2):29–34.
41. Reddoch KM, Pidcoke HF, Montgomery RK, et al. Hemostatic function of apheresis platelets stored at 4 degrees C and 22 degrees C. Shock 2014;41(Suppl 1):54–61.
42. Rock G, Sherring VA, Tittley P. 5-day storage of platelet concentrates. Transfusion 1984;24(2):147–52.
43. Inaba K, Branco BC, Rhee P, et al. Impact of the duration of platelet storage in critically ill trauma patients. J Trauma 2011;71(6):1766–73 [discussion: 1773–4].

44. Friedmann AM, Sengul H, Lehmann H, et al. Do basic laboratory tests or clinical observations predict bleeding in thrombocytopenic oncology patients? Transfus Med Rev 2002;16(1):34–45.

45. Josephson CD, Granger S, Assmann SF, et al. Bleeding risks are higher in children versus adults given prophylactic platelet transfusions for treatment-induced hypoproliferative thrombocytopenia. Blood 2012;120(4):748–60.

46. Slichter SJ, Kaufman RM, Assmann SF, et al. Dose of prophylactic platelet transfusions and prevention of hemorrhage. N Engl J Med 2010;362(7):600–13.

47. Uhl L, Assmann SF, Hamza TH, et al. Laboratory predictors of bleeding and the effect of platelet and RBC transfusions on bleeding outcomes in the PLADO trial. Blood 2017;130(10):1247–58.

48. Curley A, Stanworth SJ, Willoughby K, et al. Randomized trial of platelet-transfusion thresholds in Neonates. N Engl J Med 2019;380(3):242–51.

49. Baharoglu MI, Cordonnier C, Salman RAS, et al. Platelet transfusion versus standard care after acute stroke due to spontaneous cerebral haemorrhage associated with antiplatelet therapy (PATCH): a randomised, open-label, phase 3 trial. Lancet 2016;387(10038):2605–13.

50. Holcomb JB, Wade CE, Michalek JE, et al. Increased plasma and platelet to red blood cell ratios improves outcome in 466 massively transfused civilian trauma patients. Ann Surg 2008;248(3):447–56.

51. Perkins JG, Andrew CP, Spinella PC, et al. An evaluation of the impact of apheresis platelets used in the setting of massively transfused trauma patients. J Trauma 2009;66(4):S77–84.

52. Perkins JG, Cap AP, Spinella PC, et al. Comparison of platelet transfusion as fresh whole blood versus apheresis platelets for massively transfused combat trauma patients (CME). Transfusion 2011;51(2):242–52.

53. Cardenas JC, Zhang X, Fox EE, et al. Platelet transfusions improve hemostasis and survival in a substudy of the prospective, randomized PROPPR trial. Blood Adv 2018;2(14):1696–704.

54. Getz TM, Montgomery RK, Bynum JA, et al. Storage of platelets at 4 degrees C in platelet additive solutions prevents aggregate formation and preserves platelet functional responses. Transfusion 2016;56(6):1320–8.

55. Nair PM, Pidcoke HF, Cap AP, et al. Effect of cold storage on shear-induced platelet aggregation and clot strength. J Trauma Acute Care 2014;77:S88–93.

56. Egidi MG, D'Alessandro A, Mandarello G, et al. Troubleshooting in platelet storage temperature and new perspectives through proteomics. Blood Transfus 2010;8:S73–81.

57. Johnson L, Tan S, Wood B, et al. Refrigeration and cryopreservation of platelets differentially affect platelet metabolism and function: a comparison with conventional platelet storage conditions. Transfusion 2016;56(7):1807–18.

58. Reddoch KM, Montgomery RK, Rodriguez AC, et al. Endothelium-derived inhibitors efficiently attenuate the aggregation and adhesion responses of refrigerated platelets. Shock 2016;45(2):220–7.

59. Torres Filho IP, Torres LN, Valdez C, et al. Refrigerated platelets stored in whole blood up to 5 days adhere to thrombi formed during hemorrhagic hypotension in rats. J Thromb Haemost 2017;15(1):163–75.

60. Scorer TG, Sharma U, Peltier G, et al. Ticagrelor induced platelet dysfunction can be assessed under shear conditions and correction by platelets is influenced by storage temperature. Blood 2018;132:526.

61. Stolla M, Vargas A, Bailey S, et al. Cold-stored platelets to reverse dual antiplatelet therapy. Blood 2018;132:525.

62. Filip DJ, Aster RH. Relative hemostatic effectiveness of human platelets stored at 4-degrees-C and 22-degrees-C. J Lab Clin Med 1978;91(4):618–24.
63. Kahn RA, Staggs SD, Miller WV, et al. Recovery, lifespan, and function of CPD-Adenine (CPDA-1) platelet concentrates stored for up to 72 hours at 4 C. Transfusion 1980;20(5):498–503.
64. Slichter SJ, Harker LA. Preparation and storage of platelet concentrates. Transfusion 1976;16(1):8–12.
65. Strandenes G, Kristoffersen EK, Bjerkvig CK, et al. Cold stored platelets for treatment of postoperative bleeding in cardiothoracic surgery. Transfusion 2016;56(S4):16A.
66. Andrews RK, Berndt MC. Platelet physiology: in cold blood. Curr Biol 2003; 13(7):R282–4.
67. Chen WC, Liang X, Syed AK, et al. Inhibiting GPIb shedding preserves post-transfusion recovery and hemostatic function of platelets after prolonged storage. Arterioscl Throm Vas. 2016;36(9):1821–8.
68. Getz TM. Physiology of cold-stored platelets. Transfus Apher Sci 2019; 58(1):12–5.
69. Hoffmeister KM, Josefsson EC, Isaac NA, et al. Glycosylation restores survival of chilled blood platelets. Science 2003;301(5639):1531–4.
70. Quach ME, Chen WC, Li RH. Mechanisms of platelet clearance and translation to improve platelet storage. Blood 2018;131(14):1512–21.
71. Rumjantseva V, Hoffmeister KM. Novel and unexpected clearance mechanisms for cold platelets. Transfus Apher Sci 2010;42(1):63–70.
72. Bode AP, Knupp CL. Effect of cold storage on platelet glycoprotein Ib and vesiculation. Transfusion 1994;34(8):690–6.
73. Hoffmeister KM, Falet H, Toker A, et al. Mechanisms of cold-induced platelet actin assembly. J Biol Chem 2001;276(27):24751–9.
74. Li Y, Fu JX, Ling Y, et al. Sialylation on O-glycans protects platelets from clearance by liver Kupffer cells. Proc Natl Acad Sci U S A 2017;114(31):8360–5.
75. Sorensen AL, Rumjantseva V, Nayeb-Hashemi S, et al. Role of sialic acid for platelet life span: exposure of beta-galactose results in the rapid clearance of platelets from the circulation by asialoglycoprotein receptor-expressing liver macrophages and hepatocytes. Blood 2009;114(8):1645–54.
76. Manno CS, Hedberg KW, Kim HC, et al. Comparison of the hemostatic effects of fresh whole-blood, stored whole-blood, and components after open-heart-surgery in children. Blood 1991;77(5):930–6.
77. Reddoch-Cardenas KM, Montgomery RK, Lafleur CB, et al. Cold storage of platelets in platelet additive solution: an in vitro comparison of two Food and Drug Administration–approved collection and storage systems. Transfusion 2018;58(7):1682–8.
78. Hess JR. Resuscitation of trauma-induced coagulopathy. Hematology Am Soc Hematol Educ Program 2013;664–7.
79. Spinella PC, Pidcoke HF, Strandenes G, et al. Whole blood for hemostatic resuscitation of major bleeding. Transfusion 2016;56(Suppl 2):S190–202.
80. Strandenes G, Berseus O, Cap AP, et al. Low titer group O whole blood in emergency situations. Shock 2014;41(Suppl 1):70–5.
81. Heddle NM, Klama L, Singer J, et al. The role of the plasma from platelet concentrates in transfusion reactions. N Engl J Med 1994;331(10):625–8.
82. Stolla M, Refaai MA, Heal JM, et al. Platelet transfusion - the new immunology of an old therapy. Front Immunol 2015;6:28.

83. Khan SY, Kelher MR, Heal JM, et al. Soluble CD40 ligand accumulates in stored blood components, primes neutrophils through CD40, and is a potential cofactor in the development of transfusion-related acute lung injury. Blood 2006;108(7):2455–62.
84. Phipps RP, Kaufman J, Blumberg N. Platelet derived CD154 (CD40 ligand) and febrile responses to transfusion. Lancet 2001;357(9273):2023–4.
85. Kanter J, Khan SY, Kelher M, et al. Oncogenic and angiogenic growth factors accumulate during routine storage of apheresis platelet concentrates. Clin Cancer Res 2008;14(12):3942–7.
86. Kapur R, Zufferey A, Boilard E, et al. Nouvelle cuisine: platelets served with inflammation. J Immunol 2015;194(12):5579–87.
87. Kral JB, Schrottmaier WC, Salzmann M, et al. Platelet interaction with innate immune cells. Transfus Med Hemother 2016;43(2):78–88.
88. Finsterbusch M, Schrottmaier WC, Kral-Pointner JB, et al. Measuring and interpreting platelet-leukocyte aggregates. Platelets 2018;29(7):677–85.
89. Caron A, Theoret JF, Mousa SA, et al. Anti-platelet effects of GPIIb/IIIa and P-selectin antagonism, platelet activation, and binding to neutrophils. J Cardiovasc Pharmacol 2002;40(2):296–306.
90. Lam FW, Vijayan KV, Rumbaut RE. Platelets and their interactions with other immune cells. Compr Physiol 2015;5(3):1265–80.
91. Lievens D, Zernecke A, Seijkens T, et al. Platelet CD40L mediates thrombotic and inflammatory processes in atherosclerosis. Blood 2010;116(20):4317–27.
92. Hidari KI, Weyrich AS, Zimmerman GA, et al. Engagement of P-selectin glycoprotein ligand-1 enhances tyrosine phosphorylation and activates mitogen-activated protein kinases in human neutrophils. J Biol Chem 1997;272(45):28750–6.
93. Weyrich AS, Elstad MR, McEver RP, et al. Activated platelets signal chemokine synthesis by human monocytes. J Clin Invest 1996;97(6):1525–34.
94. Ayukawa O, Nakamura K, Kariyazono H, et al. Enhanced platelet responsiveness due to chilling and its relation to CD40 ligand level and platelet-leukocyte aggregate formation. Blood Coagul Fibrinolysis 2009;20(3):176–84.
95. Wu X, Darlington DN, Montgomery RK, et al. Platelets derived from fresh and cold-stored whole blood participate in clot formation in rats with acute traumatic coagulopathy. Br J Haematol 2017;179(5):802–10.
96. Gitz E, Koekman CA, van den Heuvel DJ, et al. Improved platelet survival after cold storage by prevention of glycoprotein Ibalpha clustering in lipid rafts. Haematologica 2012;97(12):1873–81.
97. Penberthy KK, Ravichandran KS. Apoptotic cell recognition receptors and scavenger receptors. Immunol Rev 2016;269(1):44–59.
98. Grau A, Tabib A, Grau I, et al. Apoptotic cells induce NF-kappaB and inflammasome negative signaling. PLoS One 2015;10(3):e0122440.
99. Voll RE, Herrmann M, Roth EA, et al. Immunosuppressive effects of apoptotic cells. Nature 1997;390(6658):350–1.
100. Mannino MH, Zhu Z, Xiao H, et al. The paradoxical role of IL-10 in immunity and cancer. Cancer Lett 2015;367(2):103–7.
101. Herzig MC, Reddoch-Cardenas K, Sharma U, et al. Cold-stored platelets are not pro-inflammatory in an in vitro mixed lymphocyte reaction. Transfusion 2018; 58:62A.

The Development and Impact of Hemostatic Stewardship Programs

Kathryn E. Dane, PharmD[a], Michael B. Streiff, MD[b],
John Lindsley, PharmD[a], Manuela Plazas Montana[b],
Satish Shanbhag, MBBS, MPH[c],*

KEYWORDS

- Stewardship • clotting factor concentrates • Hemophilia • Anticoagulation reversal
- Von Willebrand's disease

KEY POINTS

- The availability of clotting factor concentrates (CFCs) and anticoagulation antidotes is increasing.
- Clotting factor concentrates and anticoagulation antidotes are associated with high cost and complexity.
- Multidisciplinary hemostatic stewardship programs assist in CFC and anticoagulation antidote selection, dosing, and monitoring, resulting in enhanced patient care and reduction in drug costs.

Hemostatic disorders, which encompass diseases that predispose to bleeding (such as hemophilia and von Willebrand disease) and thrombosis (deep vein thrombosis, pulmonary embolism), are common causes of morbidity and mortality in the United States.[1] There has been a dramatic increase in the number of new treatments for

Disclosure Statement: Dr S. Shanbhag reports grants from Luitpold Pharma / Daiichi-Sankyo, outside the submitted work. Dr M.B. Streiff reports personal fees from Bayer, personal fees from CSL Behring, personal fees from Daiichi-Sankyo, grants from Boehringer Ingelheim, personal fees from Pfizer, grants and personal fees from Portola, grants from Roche, personal fees from Paul, Weiss, Rifkind, Wharton & Garrison LLP, personal fees from Lindell and Lavoie LLP, personal fees from Arnold Porter Kaye and Scholer LLP, personal fees from Cunningham Meyer and Vedrine, PC, personal fees from Gallagher & Kennedy, personal fees from Martinez Manglardi, P.A., outside the submitted work. Other authors report no competing interests.
[a] Department of Pharmacy, The Johns Hopkins Hospital, 600 North Wolfe Street, Carnegie Building, Suite 180, Baltimore, MD 21287, USA; [b] Division of Hematology, Department of Medicine, Johns Hopkins University School of Medicine, 1830 East Monument Street, Suite 7300, Baltimore, MD 21205, USA; [c] Division of Hematology, Department of Medicine, Johns Hopkins University School of Medicine, 4940 Eastern Avenue, 301 Building, Suite 4500, Baltimore, MD 21224, USA
* Corresponding author.
E-mail address: sshanbh2@jhmi.edu

Hematol Oncol Clin N Am 33 (2019) 887–901
https://doi.org/10.1016/j.hoc.2019.05.010
0889-8588/19/© 2019 Elsevier Inc. All rights reserved.

hemostatic disorders in the past decade (**Table 1**).[2] The purpose of this article was to review these products and highlight the potential role of a hemostatic stewardship programs in managing these expensive complex therapies in an efficient and cost-effective manner.

Until the 1960s, the treatment options for hemophilia were limited to whole blood or plasma. In 1964, Dr Judith Graham Pool discovered cryoprecipitate was a rich source of factor VIII. The development of cryoprecipitate allowed physicians to administer large doses of factor VIII in relatively small volumes to patients with hemophilia, making performance of surgery or the treatment of severe bleeding episodes feasible. In the 1970s, lyophilized factor concentrates became available, which allowed patients with hemophilia to administer clotting factor concentrates (CFCs) at home for the management of acute bleeding episodes and for primary prophylaxis. The cloning of the factor VIII and IX genes allowed for the development of recombinant factor VIII and IX products, which has helped to reduce the risk of infectious complications associated with administration of older plasma-derived products and cryoprecipitate.[3–5] Although these products have made factor prophylaxis much safer and more effective, the relatively short half-life of CFCs means that intravenous doses are necessary several times per week to prevent spontaneous bleeding episodes. Although venous access devices can reduce the inconvenience and discomfort of frequent CFC infusions, these devices are associated with an increased risk of bloodstream infections and catheter-associated venous thromboses.

The shortcomings of existing CFC replacement products and advances in biotechnology have led to the development of extended half-life factor VIII and IX products via several approaches. One tactic is to fuse the factor VIII or factor IX molecules to the Fc portion of the immunoglobulin G1 protein. Immunoglobulin G1 has a half-life of 21 days due to recycling of immunoglobulin G via the Fc receptor on the surface of endothelial cells. This strategy results in a 1.8-fold and 3-fold increase in the circulating half-life of the recombinant fusion protein compared with unmodified factor products. Another approach is to fuse the factor molecule to albumin, which has a 20-day half-life due to recycling via the neonatal Fc receptor. This approach increases the circulating half-life of a factor IX fusion protein by fourfold to fivefold. The third method involves fusion of factor molecules to polyethylene glycol (PEG), a polymer composed of variable numbers of ethylene oxide subunits. These approaches allow patients with hemophilia A and B to administer prophylactic doses as infrequently as every 3 to 4 days and 7 to 10 days, respectively.[6–8]

HEMOSTATIC STEWARDSHIP PROGRAMS: HISTORY AND PROGRAM DEVELOPMENT

Due to the high cost of CFCs and anticoagulation antidotes, risk of treatment-associated adverse events, and narrow therapeutic window, there has been increasing interest in identifying methods to optimize utilization of these agents and curtail drug costs. Although the concept of drug-related stewardship is relatively new to hematology, antimicrobial stewardship (AMS) programs have been in place since the mid-1990s[9] and are now recommended by the Centers for Disease Control and Prevention as an essential service for all acute care hospitals in the United States.[10] AMS programs have demonstrated improved patient outcomes and concomitant reductions in medication expenditures.[11,12] Considering the successes of AMS programs, the development of hemostatic stewardship programs has become increasingly prevalent. Although the specific medication-focus differs, the core tenants required to establish successful hemostatic stewardship programs are the

Table 1
Clotting factor concentrate products

Product (Manufacturer)	Properties	Mean Half-Life, h	Average Wholesale Price, USD
Standard half-life factor VIII products			
Advate (Shire, Lexington, MA, USA)	Recombinant full-length factor VIII	12	$1.97 per unit
Afstyla (CSL Behring, King of Prussia, PA, USA)[a]	Recombinant single-chain B-domain truncated factor VIII	14.2	$1.98 unit
Helixate FS (CSL Behring)	Recombinant full-length factor VIII	13.7–14.6	$1.76 per unit
Hemofil M (Shire)	Pooled human plasma-derived factor VIII	14.8	$1.66 per unit
Kogenate FS (Bayer, Leverkusen, Germany)	Recombinant full-length factor VIII	13.7–14.6	$1.97 per unit
Kovaltry (Bayer)	Recombinant full-length factor VIII	14	$2.12 per unit
NovoEight (Novo Nordisk)	Recombinant B-domain truncated factor VIII	11–12	$2.18 per unit
Nuwiq (Octopharma, Hoboken, NJ, USA)	Recombinant B-domain deleted factor VIII	17.1	$2.03 per unit
Recombinate (Shire)	Recombinant full-length factor VIII	14.6 ± 4.9	$1.97 per unit
Xyntha (Pfizer, New York, NY, USA)	Recombinant B-domain-deleted factor VIII	11–17	$1.90 per unit
Extended half-life factor VIII products			
Adynovate (Shire)	PEGylated full-length recombinant factor VIII protein	14.7 ± 3.79	$2.63 per unit
Eloctate (Biogen, Cambridge, MA, USA)	B-domain-deleted Factor VIII-IgG1-Fc domain fusion	16.4–19.7	$2.60 per unit
Standard half-life factor IX products			
AlphaNine SD (Grifols, Barcelona, Spain)	Pooled human plasma-derived factor IX	21–25	$1.67 per unit
Benefix (Pfizer)	Recombinant full-length factor IX	11–36	$1.64 per unit
IXinity (Aptevo BioTherapeutics LLC, Seattle, WA, USA)	Recombinant full-length factor IX	13–43	$1.99 per unit
Mononine (CSL Behring)	Pooled human plasma-derived factor IX	21–25	$1.66 per unit
Rixubis (Shire)	Recombinant full-length factor IX	26	$1.86 per unit

(continued on next page)

Table 1
(continued)

Product (Manufacturer)	Properties	Mean Half-Life, h	Average Wholesale Price, USD
Extended half-life factor IX products			
Alprolix (Biogen)[b]	Recombinant factor IX-IgG1 Fc fusion protein	87	$3.74 per unit
Idelvion (CSL Behring)[c]	Recombinant factor IX-albumin fusion protein	104–118	$5.28 per unit
Rebinyn (Novo Nordisk)[d]	Recombinant factor IX conjugated to 40 kDa polyethylene glycol	83	$4.94 per unit
Von Willebrand factor products			
Humate-P (CSL Behring)	VWF:FVIII ratio = 2.4:1	VWF: 3–34	$1.57 per RCo unit
Wilate (Octapharma)	VWF:FVIII ratio = 1:1	VWF: 6–49	$1.68 per RCo unit
Vonvendi (Shire)	Contains no FVIII	19–22.6	$2.38 per RCo unit
Other CFCs			
NovoSeven RT (Novo Nordisk)	Recombinant human factor VIIa	2.8–3.1	$2.69 per μg
Kcentra (CSL Behring)	Plasma-derived 4-factor inactivated prothrombin complex concentrate	6–8	$2.90 per unit
FEIBA (Shire)	Plasma-derived 4-factor activated prothrombin complex concentrate	4–7	$2.17 per unit
Thrombate III (Grifols)	Plasma-derived human antithrombin-III	3.8 d[e]	$4.66 per unit

Abbreviations: CFC, clotting factor concentrate; FIX, factor IX; FVIII, factor VIII; RCo, ristocetin cofactor; VWF, von Willebrand factor.
[a] Chromogenic factor VIII assay preferred for monitoring (1-stage factor VIII assay underestimates factor activity by 50%).
[b] Use of a kaolin-based activated partial thromboplastin time (aPTT) reagent for factor IX assay has been shown to underestimate factor IX levels with this CFC.
[c] Use of kaolin-based aPTT reagents or reagents insensitive to lupus inhibitors underestimates factor IX levels by 50% with this CFC.
[d] Chromogenic factor IX assay recommended or a 1-stage aPTT assay validated for use with this CFC (Silica-based aPTT reagents overestimate factor IX levels with this CFC).
[e] Half-life may be shorter following surgery, during acute thrombosis or heparin therapy.
Data from Lexicomp Online. Lexi-Drugs. Hudson: Wolters Kluwer Clinical Drug Information, Inc.; 2019.

same as those guiding AMS programs (**Fig. 1**).[10] Application of the core elements of stewardship serves as a backbone for successful stewardship program development.

Several institutions have reported significant reductions in medication expenditure with the implementation of hemostatic stewardship programs (**Table 2**).[13–16] Although the structure of each program and targeted interventions varied slightly, each program provided focused oversight of patient selection, dosing, and monitoring of select CFCs, anticoagulation reversal agents, and intravenous direct thrombin inhibitors. Reported cost savings ranged from 14% to 59%, resulting in an absolute reduction in medication expenditure of $374,539 to $4,000,000 (USD). Although pharmacists are not acknowledged as core members of the hemophilia treatment team by available guidelines,[17,18] all 4 programs reported clinical pharmacist involvement, with 2 described as pharmacist-led. Pharmacist involvement in hemostatic stewardship programs improves the medication utilization process, increases the continuity of care on inpatient care teams, and may improve adherence to hospital-specific clinical guidelines when available. Based on the core elements of stewardship and reported success of hemostatic stewardship programs, a stewardship program was developed at our institution co-led by 2 clinical pharmacists and 2 adult hematology attending physicians. The initial targeted interventions of our program include the following:

1. Formulary management of CFCs and institutional clinical guideline development
2. Continuous-infusion CFC administration
3. Recombinant factor VIIa (NovoSeven) dose minimization
4. Reduction in inappropriate antithrombin-III (AT) use
5. Fixed-dose administration of 4-factor prothrombin complex concentrate (PCC) products
6. Andexanet alfa stewardship
7. Preferential use of factor VIII inhibitor bypassing activity (FEIBA) over recombinant factor VIIa for patients with hemophilia with inhibitors

Herein, the authors describe supporting data and implementation considerations for several of these interventions.

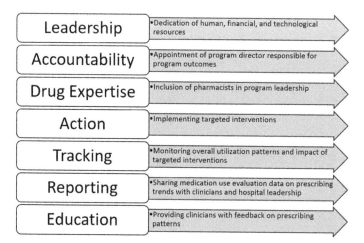

Leadership • Dedication of human, financial, and technological resources

Accountability • Appointment of program director responsible for program outcomes

Drug Expertise • Inclusion of pharmacists in program leadership

Action • Implementing targeted interventions

Tracking • Monitoring overall utilization patterns and impact of targeted interventions

Reporting • Sharing medication use evaluation data on prescribing trends with clinicians and hospital leadership

Education • Providing clinicians with feedback on prescribing patterns

Fig. 1. Core elements of stewardship. (*Data from* Centers for Disease Control and Prevention (CDC). Core Elements of Hospital Antibiotic Stewardship Programs, 2015. Available at: https://www.cdc.gov/antibiotic-use/healthcare/implementation/core-elements.html. Accessed Feb 3 2019.)

Table 2
Impact of established hemostatic and antithrombotic stewardship programs

Institution	Program Structure	Focused Interventions	Prestewardship Program Annual Clotting Factor Cost, USD	Savings, %
The University of North Carolina Medical Center[13]	• Pharmacist-led in conjunction with benign hematologists	• Institutional clinical guideline implementation • Formulary product reevaluation and selection of one formulary product per therapeutic class • Preferential use of FEIBA over NovoSeven for patients with hemophilia with inhibitors • Conversion from intermittent bolus administration of factor VIII and IX products to continuous infusion • Dose minimization for off-label NovoSeven administration	$7,900,000	>$4,000,000 (50%)
Brigham and Women's Hospital[14]	• Led by Hematology Medical Director • Involvement with pharmacists and inpatient hematology attending physicians	• Reduction in NovoSeven utilization for patients with hemophilia with inhibitors • Reduction in intravenous direct thrombin inhibitor use	$10,247,104	$1,449,417 (14%)
Indiana University Health[15]	• Clinical pharmacist led	• Reduction in off-label NovoSeven and Profilnine-SD administration via prospective review of all orders by clinical pharmacist pursuant to clinical guideline	$505,684	$374,539 (14%)
Rush University Medical Center[16]	• Clinical pharmacist in conjunction with benign hematologists and Hemophilia Treatment Center Team	• Formulary management of CFCs • Establishment of 340B account for CFC use in outpatient areas • Clinical management of hemophilia patients	$4,600,000	$2,700,000 (59%)

Abbreviation: CFC, clotting factor concentrate.

FORMULARY MANAGEMENT OF CLOTTING FACTOR CONCENTRATES AND INSTITUTIONAL CLINICAL GUIDELINE DEVELOPMENT

An early priority in the development of our stewardship program was to critically reevaluate our formulary CFC products. As a part of this process, a thorough medication use evaluation was conducted for each therapeutic class to identify utilization patterns and areas for improvement. Our aim was to ensure only the most cost-effective products were on the formulary, and to limit the number of formulary options within each therapeutic class. Although there are an increasing number of CFC products available with the advent of extended half-life factor VIII and IX products, extended half-life products offer no additional advantage over standard half-life products for inpatients, and are generally associated with increased cost. When evaluating formulary options for each CFC therapeutic class, we considered the following factors: inhibitor formation risk (for factor VIII products only), availability of extended stability data allowing for continuous-infusion administration (factor VIII, IX, and von Willebrand factor products), and cost. With these considerations, we consolidated available factor VIII formulary options from 6 to 2 products, and factor IX products from 3 to 1 product. Similar to reported outcomes from other hemostatic stewardship programs, we anticipate significant cost savings as a result of these formulary changes.[13]

To assist in optimizing patient selection, dosing, and monitoring of CFCs, we have also developed institutional clinical guidelines for utilization of CFCs and anticoagulation antidotes. These guidelines contain both drug modules and disease state modules. Drug modules provide information on restriction status, acceptable and unacceptable uses, pharmacokinetics and pharmacodynamics, dosing, monitoring, drug interactions, adverse effects, and links to relevant hospital policies. Disease state modules consist of similar dosing recommendations to drug modules, but also address diagnostic considerations and choice of therapy. These guidelines will be made available to all clinicians at our institution to promote consistency in CFC and anticoagulation antidote utilization patterns.

CONTINUOUS-INFUSION CLOTTING FACTOR CONCENTRATE ADMINISTRATION

The goal of CFC replacement is to maintain the minimal factor activity level required for normal hemostasis. To achieve this, CFCs have been historically administered as intermittent boluses every 8 to 24 hours to maintain the desired trough level. However, this approach necessitates administering a large factor dose that achieves a supraphysiologic peak to ensure factor levels remain above the intended trough level. Continuous-infusion CFC administration overcomes this limitation by minimizing peak-trough factor level fluctuations, which increases the time above the desired factor level and reduces factor consumption and cost by as much as 30%.[19] Increased time above the desired factor level with continuous-infusion CFC administration has translated to improved efficacy, with reported reductions in postoperative transfusion requirements for surgical patients and higher hemoglobin levels.[19]

Historically, concerns regarding the safety of CFC administration via continuous infusion included infectious risk, thrombophlebitis, and an increased risk of inhibitor formation. Initial concerns about the stability and infectious risk of CFCs when reconstituted for more than a few hours have not been substantiated.[20] Experts advise that factor products for continuous infusion should be administered as concentrated product and not be further diluted. Although thrombophlebitis was noted in early studies of continuous-infusion CFC, the addition of unfractionated heparin (5 units/mL) administration via central line, or infusion in parallel with saline (20 mL/h) has largely eliminated this issue. Although some studies have noted an increased incidence of factor inhibitors associated with continuous-infusion CFCs, a prospective study of continuous-infusion therapy limited to patients with 50 or more exposure days did not note any inhibitor development.[21] Therefore, factor inhibitor risk may not be associated with use of continuous-infusion therapy, but rather intensive CFC administration in patients with limited previous treatment exposures.[20,22]

In light of the advantages of continuous-infusion CFC therapy for management of surgery or major bleeds, many centers in Europe use continuous-infusion therapy. In preparation for elective surgery, centers often conduct pharmacokinetic testing to determine optimal factor infusion rates. All respondents to the European survey used factor concentrates without additional dilution and used syringe pumps or mini-pumps for infusions. Heparin (5 units/mL) added to the concentrate or parallel infusions of saline were used to reduce the risk of local thrombophlebitis by some centers. Generally, centers target factor levels 80% to 100% during surgery and 50% to 80% during the first 3 postoperative days. Thereafter, factor levels 40% to 80% are targeted. Most centers adjusted factor infusions using daily factor levels. Thrombophlebitis occurred in 2% to 11% of patients and no infections were reported. Eight centers (89%) reported cost savings with continuous-infusion CFCs over bolus administration, with estimated savings ranging from 15% to 36%. Factor inhibitors were reported in 9 of 742 patients (1.2%) and almost exclusively occurred in patients with fewer than 50 treatment days. All centers reported good to excellent hemostasis with this approach.[22]

Due to the known benefits of CFC administration via continuous infusion, we believe this administration strategy should be strongly considered for patients receiving factor VIII, IX, or von Willebrand factor concentrates undergoing major surgery or with severe bleeding presentations. In addition to the principles outlined previously, to safely deliver continuous-infusion therapy, several precautions should be implemented before executing CFC administration via continuous infusion. Formulary CFC products should be reevaluated for extended stability to ensure product integrity with infusion durations of 12 hours or more. On admission, required actions to ensure a dedicated line is available for continuous-infusion CFC administration should be standardized. The compatibility of available infusion pumps with the necessary drug delivery volume must be considered. As a result of the consequences of interruptions in continuous-infusion CFC administration for postoperative patients or those with severe bleeds, multidisciplinary education should occur before implementation. Due to infrequent administration at many centers, reeducation should take place with every new initiation. A multidisciplinary team is necessary to ensure the previously described steps are considered for every patient receiving continuous-infusion CFC replacement.

RECOMBINANT FACTOR VIIa (NovoSeven) DOSE MINIMIZATION

Recombinant coagulation factor VIIa (rVIIa; NovoSeven) is approved by the Food and Drug Administration (FDA) for the treatment of rare bleeding diatheses, including congenital hemophilia with inhibitors, acquired hemophilia, Glanzmann thrombasthenia, and congenital factor VII deficiency. However, it has been studied extensively for off-label administration to manage severe bleeding or prophylactically to prevent operative blood loss in other populations (eg, perioperative bleeding, intracranial hemorrhage, postpartum hemorrhage, trauma) with largely disappointing results.[23] A Cochrane review concluded that the effectiveness of rFVIIa as a general hemostatic drug (outside of hemophilia) was unproven, and patients receiving rFVIIa had an increased risk of arterial thromboembolic events. The use of rFVIIa for off-label indications persists despite the lack of randomized clinical trial data supporting its use and multiple systematic reviews and meta-analyses showing no mortality benefit.[24] Also, rVIIa administration is associated with substantial cost ($18,830 [USD] for 90 µg/kg dose in an 80-kg individual) and can require dosing as frequently as every 2 hours.

Administration of rVIIa to manage postoperative bleeding in cardiac surgery accounts for most off-label use at our institution. Observational data in this population suggest no difference in bleeding response or 28-day mortality with low-dose rVIIa (≤40 µg/kg, median 27 µg/kg) compared with high-dose (52 µg/kg–109 µg/kg).[25] In addition, observational studies have demonstrated a significant reduction in surgical reexploration, 24-hour blood loss, and transfusion requirements with rVIIa doses as low as 17 µg/kg when compared with propensity matched controls.[26] Using lower doses of rVIIa (17–30 µg/kg) when administered for life-threatening bleeding following cardiac surgery has the potential to limit the adverse effect profile without impacting efficacy.[27]

Stewardship of rVIIa ensures rapid access to a life-saving drug for approved indications, while restricting inappropriate use. Outside of FDA-approved indications, we restrict rVIIa for management of critical bleeding refractory to anticoagulation reversal (if applicable), and antifibrinolytics, despite normalization of coagulation parameters, and failure of surgical attempts to control bleeding. The efficacy of rVIIa is reduced by 90% in the setting of acidosis with pH <7.1 and by 20% when administered to patients with a core body temperature of 33°C.[28] Therefore, attempts to normalize pH and hypothermia must be under way while VIIa use is being considered. If administered for off-label indications, the lowest dose demonstrating efficacy in each specific patient population should be used in lieu of higher FDA-approved doses.

REDUCTION IN INAPPROPRIATE ANTITHROMBIN USE

Antithrombin (AT) concentrate (Thrombate) is FDA-approved for the treatment and prevention of thromboembolism in patients with hereditary AT deficiency. However, many institutions have a high prevalence of off-label AT concentrate administration for the management of heparin resistance. In a retrospective analysis of AT concentration administration, Ciolek and colleagues[29] noted that more than 50% of AT concentrate administrations were deemed inappropriate, resulting in $528,095 (USD) in unnecessary drug expenditure. The results of this evaluation have been used at our institution to begin implementation of formulary restrictions for non-intraoperative AT administration, using the appropriate use criteria in **Table 3** as the primary basis for the restriction. In addition, we have implemented guidance to define appropriate intraoperative AT administration (**Fig. 2**) to reduce unnecessary administration for adult cardiac surgeries requiring cardiopulmonary bypass. These interventions can potentially result in a significant reduction in inappropriate AT administration and substantial cost savings.

FIXED-DOSE ADMINISTRATION OF 4-FACTOR PROTHROMBIN COMPLEX CONCENTRATE PRODUCTS

PCC is a plasma-derived CFC that contains vitamin K–dependent clotting factors. PCC products are available as 3-factor (3F-PCC) or 4-factor concentrates (4F-PCC). Both PCC products contain 25 times the concentration of factors II, IX, and X found in normal human plasma, and 4F-PCC also contains factor VII.[30] Four-factor PCC is an effective agent for the reversal of vitamin K antagonists (VKAs) in the setting of hemorrhage. Available data demonstrate that a weight-based 4F-PCC dose provides more rapid and complete reversal compared with fresh frozen plasma. Although no randomized controlled trials are available directly comparing 4F-PCC with 3F-PCC for

Table 3
Criteria for determination of appropriate indications for AT

Criteria for non-ECMO patients	1. AT level drawn ≤24 h before AT repletion 2. Receiving UFH infusion 3. Subtherapeutic AT level[a] 4. Subtherapeutic UFH anti-Xa level
Criteria for ECMO patients	1. AT level drawn ≤24 h before AT repletion 2. Receiving UFH infusion 3. Subtherapeutic AT level[a] 4. Subtherapeutic UFH anti-Xa level 5. Normal fibrinogen and aPTT

Abbreviations: aPTT, activated partial thromboplastin time; AT, antithrombin; ECMO, extracorporeal membrane oxygenation; UFH, unfractionated heparin.

   [a] ≤30 days old: AT less than 50%; >30 days old: AT less than 80%.

   Adapted from Ciolek A, Lindsley J, Crow J, et al. Identification of Cost-Saving Opportunities for the Use of Antithrombin III in Adult and Pediatric Patients. Clinical and Applied Thrombosis/Hemostasis 2017;24(1):186-191; with permission.

warfarin reversal, 4F-PCC offers a theoretic advantage because it also contains factor VII and is therefore recommended as the first-line agent for VKA reversal in current guidelines.[31]

According to the FDA labeling, initial 4F-PCC dosing for VKA reversal uses patient weight and initial international normalized ratio (INR) to guide dosing (range 25 units/kg per dose to 50 units/kg per dose). The calculated dose uses the factor IX content of the product, as PCCs were originally developed for the management of hemophilia B.[30] For patients with critical VKA-induced bleeding, awaiting INR results to guide PCC dosing can lead to delays in treatment. Thus, alternative dosing strategies may promote more rapid reversal of VKA-associated bleeding. Several retrospective evaluations have explored the use of lower fixed dosing of 4F-PCC for VKA reversal (**Table 4**).[32–34] Overall, a fixed 4F-PCC dose of 1000 to 1500 units lowered the INR to an acceptable range in most patients, resulted in decreased 4F-PCC cost, and may lead to decreased thromboembolic events associated with reversal. In addition, because no baseline INR is required with this strategy before administration for patients known to be taking VKAs, decreased time to treatment was also observed. Although these findings are limited to small retrospective reviews at single centers,

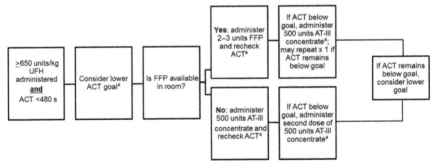

Fig. 2. Intraoperative guidance for AT administration for adult cardiac surgery. [a] Consider additional UFH bolus. ACT, activated clotting time; FFP, fresh frozen plasma.

Table 4
Summary of select fixed dosed 4F-PCC trials

Study	Design	Intervention	Baseline Characteristics	Results

Klein et al,[32] 2015	Single-center, retrospective cohort study	• 4F-PCC 1500 units fixed-dose	• 39 patients included
			• All patients had ICH as indication for reversal
			• Median age (y): 70 (IQR 60–78)
			• Median weight: 79.5 kg (IQR 72.1–95.3)
			• 71.8% presented with ICH
				• Median 4F-PCC dose: 1659 units
				• Median time to initial postadministration INR: 51 min
				• 56.7% reduction in INR
				  ○ Median INR (presentation): 3.3
				  ○ Median INR (post 4F-PCC): 1.4
				    ■ 92.3% reached INR <2
				    ■ 71.8% reached INR ≤1.5
				    ■ 2.6% received second dose for INR ≥2
				• Median costs savings
				  ○ ~$40,273 for 39 patients

Astrup et al,[33] 2018	Single-center, retrospective cohort of patients	• 4F-PCC 1500 units fixed dose	• 37 patients included
			• Indication for reversal
			  ○ 78% for emergent bleeding (45.9% ICH)
			  ○ 18.9% for urgent surgery
			• Median age (y): 70 (IQR 58–83)
			• Median weight (kg) 74.5 (IQR 61.5–83)
				• Mean 4F-PCC dose: 1601 units
				• Median time to initial INR post administration INR: 65 min (IQR 50–88)
				• Median change in INR: 1.55
				  ○ Median initial INR: 3.06
				  ○ Median INR post 4F-PCC: 1.32
				    ■ 74.3% achieved INR ≤1.5
				    ■ 100% achieved INR ≤2
				• Median cost savings of $982 per patient
				• Fixed dose led to time to decreased time to treatment 51 min (historical group) to 38 min (P = .005)

Scott et al,[34] 2018	Single-center, retrospective cohort of pre fixed-dose and post fixed-dose protocol implementation	• Fixed dosing strategy: 4F-PCC 1000 units
		• Package insert dosing strategy: 25 units/kg/dose to 50 units/kg/dose depending on patient weight and INR on presentation
			• 61 patients with ICH
			  ○ Fixed dose: 30 patients
			  ○ PI dose: 31 patients
			• Mean age (y):
			  ○ Fixed dose: 78
			  ○ PI dose: 81
			• Median weight (kg):
			  ○ Fixed dose: 82
			  ○ PI dose: 83
				• Mean dose:
				  ○ Fixed dose: 1045 units
				  ○ PI dose: 2120 units
				• Mean pre 4F-PCC INR:
				  ○ Fixed dose: 2.84
				  ○ PI: 2.98
				• INR <1.5 achieved:
				  ○ Fixed dose: 53%
				  ○ PI dose: 76% (P = .15)
				• INR <1.6 achieved:
				  ○ Fixed dose: 73%
				  ○ PI Dose: 81% (P = .49)

Abbreviations: 4F-PCC, 4-factor PCC; ICH, intracranial hemorrhage; INR, international normalized ratio; IQR, interquartile range; PI, prescribing information.

we believe this strategy is worth considering due to the promising results replicated in multiple analyses and the benefits of this approach in reducing time to reversal, adverse events, and medication cost.

ANDEXANET ALFA STEWARDSHIP

Multiple oral factor Xa inhibitors are now approved for treatment of atrial fibrillation and venous thromboembolism, with apixaban and rivaroxaban leading in market share,[35] therefore creating a need for reversal agents specific to this drug class. Although the rates of major bleeding and clinically relevant non–major bleeding for most direct oral anticoagulants (DOACs) are lower than warfarin, reversal has historically been challenging when bleeds occur due to the lack of a specific antidote.[36,37] Since the initial approval of oral factor Xa inhibitors in 2011, bleeding events on oral factor Xa inhibitors have been managed with nonspecific reversal strategies, such as activated or inactivated PCCs.[38] However, data supporting this approach are limited to clinical and laboratory observational data.

Andexanet alfa (Andexxa) is a recombinant, inactive form of factor Xa that acts as a decoy to bind and sequester factor Xa inhibitors. Through this mechanism, andexanet alfa is potentially effective in reversing any drug that works through factor Xa inhibition. However, due to limited evaluation in patients receiving edoxaban, betrixaban, enoxaparin, or fondaparinux, andexanet alfa was approved by the FDA in 2018 only for reversal of rivaroxaban and apixaban in cases of life-threatening or uncontrolled bleeding.[39]

The single-arm study prompting FDA approval included 352 patients with acute major bleeding (mostly intracranial or gastrointestinal) while on a factor Xa inhibitor. Enrolled patients received an initial bolus of andexanet alfa followed by a 2-hour infusion. Andexanet alfa administration markedly reduced anti–factor Xa activity, and 82% of patients had excellent or good hemostatic efficacy. However, the 30-day death rate was 14% and a thrombotic event was seen in 10% of patients on study. Reduction in anti–factor Xa activity was not predictive of hemostatic efficacy overall, but was modestly predictive in patients with intracranial hemorrhage.[39] Andexanet alfa dosing is based on the dose of the factor Xa inhibitor and the duration since last exposure. The cost of a single bolus and 2-hour infusion is either $29,700 (USD) or $59,400 (USD) depending the dose.[2] These factors raise significant concerns about andexanet alfa use:

- Patients may not be responsive and able to communicate which anticoagulant they are taking and/or time of last ingestion.
- Readily available coagulation tests, such as prothrombin time and activated partial thromboplastin time, are not sensitive to the presence of oral factor Xa inhibitors. Plasma anti-Xa levels must be calibrated to each oral factor Xa inhibitor, and are not rapidly available at most centers for the urgent or emergent management of active bleeding.
- There are significant thrombotic risks and major cost considerations with andexanet alfa, and the lack of a comparator arm makes the assessment of the long-term clinical benefit of this medication challenging.

From a stewardship standpoint, our goals are to ensure that patients with life-threatening bleeds have rapid access to andexanet alfa while minimizing inappropriate use. Andexanet alfa has not been studied in patients who have already received PCCs or rVIIa, and we therefore do not use it in this setting without evidence of inadequate hemostasis and confirmation of ongoing drug exposure. We allow expedited use for patients with intracranial hemorrhage associated with apixaban, rivaroxaban, or edoxaban last administered within 24 hours in the setting of a Glasgow Coma Scale ≥ 5 (a more liberal designation than the >7 cutoff in the phase III trial). We request an anti-Xa assay calibrated for unfractionated heparin (UFH) be sent before administration for all patients receiving andexanet alfa, but administration of the drug is not delayed for the result. In cases in which the last factor Xa inhibitor dose is unknown or greater than 24 hours before presentation, a UFH anti-Xa should be evaluated before andexanet administration. If the UFH anti-Xa is undetectable (<0.1 IU/mL), andexanet alfa administration is not warranted due to clinically insignificant concentrations of the factor Xa inhibitor. This test was chosen for its sensitivity to clinically significant drug levels and its rapid turnaround time of 30 minutes at our institution. Quantitative assessment of factor Xa inhibitor concentrations (rivaroxaban-specific and apixaban-specific anti-Xa assays) are available at our institution, but the results are not available in sufficient time to guide clinical decision-making.

Andexanet alfa is a novel drug with very limited supply. Smaller centers may not be able to stock a cost-prohibitive drug that is not offered on consignment. In a center in which andexanet alfa is not available, crucial time may be lost during transportation to a referral center stocking the drug. In these cases, and for patients not meeting the criteria for andexanet alfa administration at our institution, administration of activated or inactivated PCCs and other supportive measures should be considered.

SUMMARY

With increasing availability of CFCs and anticoagulation antidotes, the complexity and cost of care for patients with hemostatic disorders will continue to rise. Hemostatic stewardship programs have proven successful in CFC and anticoagulation antidote selection, dosing, and monitoring, resulting in enhanced patient care and reduction in drug costs. Potential targeted interventions for hemostatic stewardship programs include CFC formulary management and institutional clinical guideline development; rVIIa, AT, and 4F-PCC dose minimization; reduction in inappropriate AT use; preferential use of FEIBA over rVIIa for patients with hemophilia with inhibitors; and andexanet alfa stewardship. To effectively implement a cohesive hemostatic stewardship program, a multidisciplinary team consisting of physician and pharmacist leadership should be assembled with support from hospital leadership. Ongoing assessment of CFC and antidote utilization and education are essential for program success.

REFERENCES

1. Beckman MG, Hooper WC, Critchley SE, et al. Venous thromboembolism: a public health concern. Am J Prev Med 2010;38(4):S495–501.
2. Lexicomp online, Lexi drugs online. Hudson (OH): Wolters Kluwer Clinical Drug Information, Inc; 2019. Available at: http://www.crlonline.com/lco/action/home. Accessed February 10, 2019.
3. Franchini M, Mannucci P. Past, present and future of hemophilia: a narrative review. Orphanet J Rare Dis 2012;7(1):24.
4. Morfini M, Coppola A, Franchini M, et al. Clinical use of factor VIII and factor IX concentrates. Blood Transfus 2013;11(Suppl 4):s55–63.
5. Medical and Scientific Advisory Council (MASAC) of the National Hemophilia Foundation (NHF). Products Licensed in the U.S. to Treat HEMOPHILIA. 2018. Available at: https://www.hemophilia.org/sites/default/files/document/files/253 Tables.pdf. Accessed February 7, 2019.
6. Powell JS. Longer-acting clotting factor concentrates for hemophilia. J Thromb Haemost 2015;13(Suppl 1):s167–75.

7. Cafuir LA, Kempton CL. Current and emerging factor VIII replacement products for hemophilia A. Ther Adv Hematol 2017;8(10):303–13.
8. Graf L. Extended half-life factor VIII and factor IX preparations. Transfus Med Hemother 2018;45(2):86–91.
9. McGowan JE Jr, Gerding DN. Does antibiotic restriction prevent resistance? New Horiz 1996;4(3):370–6.
10. Centers for Disease Control and Prevention. Core Elements of Hospital Antibiotic Stewardship Programs. 2015. Available at: https://www.cdc.gov/antibiotic-use/healthcare/implementation/core-elements.html. Accessed February 3, 2019.
11. Schuts EC, Hulscher MEJL, Mouton JW, et al. Current evidence on hospital antimicrobial stewardship objectives: a systematic review and meta-analysis. Lancet Infect Dis 2016;16(7):847–56.
12. Standiford HC, Chan S, Tripoli M, et al. Antimicrobial stewardship at a large tertiary care academic medical center: cost analysis before, during, and after a 7-year program. Infect Control Hosp Epidemiol 2012;33(4):338–45.
13. Amerine LB, Chen SL, Daniels R, et al. Impact of an innovative blood factor stewardship program on drug expense and patient care. Am J Health Syst Pharm 2015;72(18):1579–84.
14. Reardon DP, Atay JK, Ashley SW, et al. Implementation of a hemostatic and antithrombotic stewardship program. J Thromb Thrombolysis 2015;40:379–82.
15. Trueg AO, Lowe C, Kiel PJ. Clinical outcomes of a pharmacy-led blood factor stewardship program. Am J Ther 2017;24(6):e643–7.
16. Slocum GW, Peksa GD, Webb TA, et al. Implementation of a hemophilia management program improves clinical outcomes. J Am Coll Clin Pharm 2019;2:236–42.
17. National Hemophilia Foundation. Comprehensive medical care: HTCs. 2018. Available at: https://www.hemophilia.org/Researchers-Healthcare-Providers/Comprehensive-Medical-Care-Hemophilia-Treatment-Centers. Accessed February 3, 2019.
18. National Hemophilia Foundation. Standards and criteria for the care of persons with congenital bleeding disorders. 2012. Available at: https://www.hemophilia.org/Researchers-Healthcare-Providers/Medical-and-Scientific-Advisory-Council-MASAC/MASAC-Recommendations/Standards-and-Criteria-for-the-Care-of-Persons-with-Congenital-Bleeding-Disorders. Accessed February 3, 2019.
19. Batorova A, Martinowitz U. Intermittent injections vs. continuous infusion of factor VIII in haemophilia patients undergoing major surgery. Br J Haematol 2000;110(3):715–20.
20. Holme PA, Tjønnfjord GE, Batorova A. Continuous infusion of coagulation factor concentrates during intensive treatment. Haemophilia 2018;24(1):24–32.
21. Auerswald G, Bade A, Haubold K, et al. No inhibitor development after continuous infusion of factor concentrates in subjects with bleeding disorders undergoing surgery: a prospective study. Haemophilia 2013;19(3):438–44.
22. Batorova A, Holme P, Gringeri A, et al. Continuous infusion in haemophilia: current practice in Europe. Haemophilia 2012;18(5):753–9.
23. Simpson E, Lin Y, Stanworth S, et al. Recombinant factor VIIa for the prevention and treatment of bleeding in patients without haemophilia. Cochrane Database Syst Rev 2012;(3):CD005011.
24. Hsia CC, Chin-Yee IH, McAlister VC. Use of recombinant activated factor VII in patients without hemophilia: a meta-analysis of randomized control trials. Ann Surg 2008;248(1):61–8.
25. Willis C, Bird R, Mullany D, et al. Use of rFVIIa for critical bleeding in cardiac surgery: dose variation and patient outcomes. Vox Sang 2010;98(4):531–7.

26. Gelsomino S, Lorusso R, Romagnoli S, et al. Treatment of refractory bleeding after cardiac operations with low-dose recombinant activated factor VII (NovoSeven): a propensity score analysis. Eur J Cardiothorac Surg 2008;33(1):64–71.

27. Stefano Romagnoli S, Bevilacqua S, Gelsomino S, et al. Small-dose recombinant activated factor VII (NovoSeven®) in cardiac surgery. Anesth Analg 2006;102(5): 1320–6.

28. Meng ZH, Wolberg AS, Monroe DM 3rd, et al. The effect of temperature and pH on the activity of factor VIIa: implications for the efficacy of high-dose factor VIIa in hypothermic and acidotic patients. J Trauma 2003;55(5):886–91.

29. Ciolek A, Lindsley J, Crow J, et al. Identification of cost-saving opportunities for the use of antithrombin III in adult and pediatric patients. Clin Appl Thromb Hemost 2017;24(1):186–91.

30. Franchini M, Lippi G. Prothrombin complex concentrates: an update. Blood Transfus 2010;8(3):149–54.

31. Frontera JA, Lewin JJ 3rd, Rabinstein AA, et al. Guideline for reversal of antithrombotics in intracranial hemorrhage: a statement for healthcare professionals from the neurocritical care society and society of critical care medicine. Neurocrit Care 2016;24(1):6–46.

32. Klein L, Peters J, Miner J, et al. Evaluation of fixed dose 4-factor prothrombin complex concentrate for emergent warfarin reversal. Am J Emerg Med 2015; 33(9):1213–8.

33. Astrup G, Sarangarm P, Burnett A. Fixed dose 4-factor prothrombin complex concentrate for the emergent reversal of warfarin: a retrospective analysis. J Thromb Thrombolysis 2018;45(2):300–5.

34. Scott R, Kersten B, Basior J, et al. Evaluation of fixed-dose four-factor prothrombin complex concentrate for emergent warfarin reversal in patients with intracranial hemorrhage. J Emerg Med 2018;54(6):861–6.

35. Helfand C. Pfizer, BMS' Eliquis takes J&J's next-gen anticoagulant market-share crown. 2017. Available at: https://www.fiercepharma.com/marketing/pfizer-bms-eliquis-takes-j-j-s-next-gen-anticoagulant-market-share-crown. Accessed February 10, 2019.

36. Yeh CH, Gross PL, Weitz JI. Evolving use of new oral anticoagulants for treatment of venous thromboembolism. Blood 2014;124(7):1020–8.

37. Inohara T, Xian Y, Liang L, et al. Association of intracerebral hemorrhage among patients taking non-vitamin K antagonist vs vitamin K antagonist oral anticoagulants with in-hospital mortality. JAMA 2018;319(5):463–73.

38. Samuelson BT, Cuker A. Measurement and reversal of the direct oral anticoagulants. Blood Rev 2017;31(1):77–84.

39. Connolly SJ, Crowther M, Eikelboom JW, et al. Full study report of andexanet alfa for bleeding associated with factor Xa inhibitors. N Engl J Med 2019;380(14): 1326–35.

Transfusion Management in Pediatric Oncology Patients

Marianne E. Nellis, MD, MS[a],*, Ruchika Goel, MD, MPH[b,c], Oliver Karam, MD, PhD[d]

KEYWORDS

- Transfusion • Patient blood management • Children • Oncology

KEY POINTS

- In pediatric oncology patients, red blood cell transfusions should be considered if the hemoglobin level is below 7 to 8 g/dL.
- In pediatric oncology patients, platelet transfusions should be considered if the platelet count is below 10×10^9/L, or if the patient has clinically significant bleeding.
- In pediatric oncology patients, plasma transfusions should be considered if the international normalized ratio is above 2.5 and the patient has clinically significant bleeding.

BLOOD CELL TRANSFUSIONS

Physiology

Pediatric oncology patients may become anemic due to the suppression or dysfunction of erythrogenesis secondary to the underlying condition, as well as a consequence of bleeding. The balance between the tolerance to anemia and the need for transfusion may be different from other patients, due to underlying disease, the presence of comorbidities that influence the tolerance to anemia (hypoxemia), and complications of multiple previous transfusions.

Oxygen delivery (DO_2) is the product of cardiac output (CO), hemoglobin level (Hb), and arterial oxygen saturation (SaO_2), in addition to dissolved oxygen (proportional to the arterial partial pressure of oxygen [Pa_{O_2}]):

$$DO_2 = CO \times ([1.39 \times Hb \times SaO_2] + [0.03 \times Pa_{O_2}])$$

Disclosure Statement: The authors have nothing to disclose.
[a] Division of Pediatric Critical Care Medicine, Department of Pediatrics, NY Presbyterian Hospital - Weill Cornell Medicine, 525 East 68th Street, M-508, New York, NY 10065, USA; [b] Division of Hematology/Oncology, Simmons Cancer Institute at SIU School of Medicine, 315 West Carpenter Street, Springfield, IL 62702, USA; [c] Department of Pathology, Johns Hopkins University, Baltimore, MD, USA; [d] Division of Pediatric Critical Care Medicine, Department of Pediatrics, Children's Hospital of Richmond at VCU, 1250 East Marshall Street, Richmond, VA 23298, USA
* Corresponding author.
E-mail address: man9026@med.cornell.edu
; @mnellismd (M.E.N.); @ruchika_goel1 (R.G.); @DrOliverKaram (O.K.)

When the Hb level is low, some compensatory mechanisms exist to preserve DO_2:

- Decreased afterload: low Hb levels decrease the blood viscosity, which decreases the cardiac afterload, which in turn increases the CO, which increases the DO_2.[1]
- Increased stroke volume and heart rate: anemia, especially with concomitant hypovolemia, will lead to sympathetic activation, which increases stroke volume and heart rate, which in turn increases the CO, which increases the DO_2.

In addition, there are compensatory mechanisms to preserve oxygen consumption (Vo_2):

- Blood redistribution: blood is redistributed to tissues with high metabolic demands (eg, heart, brain).
- Increased oxygen extraction: low partial pressures of O_2 increase the red blood cell (RBC) production of 2,3-diphosphoglycerate (2,3 DPG), which promotes offloading of O_2 to the tissues by shifting the oxyhemoglobin dissociation curve rightward.

Observational adult studies have shown an association between anemia and poor patient outcomes in the critically ill.[2] However, there is an abundance of evidence that RBC transfusions in themselves are independently associated with worse outcomes in both adults and children.[3–5]

Indications

National audits of pediatric RBC transfusions in the United Kingdom have reported that more than half of pediatric transfusions on non-neonatal wards were given to hematology/oncology patients.[6] The most recent RBC transfusion recommendations come from the Transfusion and Anemia Expert Initiative.[7] A panel of 38 international experts developed evidence-based recommendations, based on a systematic review of more than 19,000 abstracts of which 45 articles were retained for inclusion. Although the recommendations were focused on critically ill children, it seems reasonable to also apply them to less sick patients.

In children with oncologic diagnoses or in patients undergoing hematopoietic stem cell transplantation who are critically ill or at risk for critical illness and hemodynamically stable, they suggest an Hb concentration of 7 to 8 g/dL be considered a threshold for RBC transfusion. There is a paucity of studies specific to pediatric oncology patients. A single-center study of 66 children with hematopoietic stem cell transplantation managed with a restrictive threshold of 7 g/dL was compared with a historic control group in which a threshold hemoglobin of 9 g/dL was used.[8] Postintervention, median pretransfusion Hb significantly decreased from 8.8 g/dL to 6.8 g/dL; no difference was found in length of stay, engraftment, or 100-day mortality.

Dosing

RBC transfusions are usually dosed as 10 to 15 mL/kg. In adults, it is now recommended to give one unit at a time and reassess the need for further transfusions.[9] In adults with hematologic malignancies, a single-unit RBC transfusion strategy has been shown to be safe.[10] Therefore, we would suggest transfusing 10 to 15 mL/kg, up to one unit in children.

On the other hand, although uncommonly used, the dose can be calculated (in milliliters) based on the current hemoglobin of the child, the desired hemoglobin following transfusion, and the blood volume of the child. Typically, the blood volume is 80 mL/kg if the child is younger than 2 years and 70 mL/kg if the child is 2 to 14 years old. Another factor in this calculation is the hemoglobin of the unit transfused (which can be obtained from the blood bank and is usually approximately 20 g/dL):

$$\text{Dose of RBC Transfusion} = ([Hb_{targeted} - Hb_{observed}] \times \text{Weight} \times \text{Blood Volume})/Hb_{RBC\ unit}$$

Product-Specific Considerations

Leukoreduction
Leukoreduction is one of the most common modifications to cellular blood products with universal leukoreduction being accepted increasingly as a standard. Leukoreduction can be performed either prestorage, that is, within 72 hours of collection, or pre-transfusion at the bedside. Residual leukocyte content should be less than 5.0×10^6 white blood cells per unit.[11] Leukoreduction leads to decreased febrile nonhemolytic transfusion reactions[12,13]; reduces the risk of transfusion-transmitted cytomegalovirus infection (CMV); and reduces the risk of HLA alloimmunization. Transmission of CMV by transfusion may be of concern specifically in low-birthweight ($\leq$1200 g) premature infants born to CMV-seronegative mothers and as hematopoietic progenitor cell or solid organ transplant patients, if they are CMV seronegative. The risk of CMV transmission by cellular components can be reduced by transfusing CMV-seronegative or leukocyte-reduced components. Although leukoreduced products are considered CMV safe, that is, equivalent if products from CMV-seronegative donors are unavailable, it is important to note that leukocyte reduction is not a substitute for irradiation (see discussion in the next section), which can be a prerequisite for some pediatric bone marrow transplant and some oncology patients.

Irradiation
Blood components with viable lymphocytes may need to be irradiated. The gamma irradiation prevents T-lymphocytes from proliferating and reduces the risk of transfusion-associated graft-versus-host disease (TA-GVHD), a rare but largely fatal complication in immunocompromised patients including fetuses requiring intrauterine transfusions, premature neonates, patients with cellular immunodeficiencies (eg, severe combined immunodeficiency, DiGeorge syndrome), patients with significant immunosuppression from chemotherapy (eg, use of purine analogs), immunomodulators, radiation, or hematopoietic stem cell transplant patients. Thus, irradiation is required processing for most pediatric oncology patients. It also helps prevent TA-GVHD in immunocompetent patients receiving blood products from blood relatives, directed donors, or products selected for HLA compatibility.[14] Irradiation involves gamma irradiation with 2500 cGy to the central portion of the product and a minimum of 1500 cGy to all other areas. However, irradiation damages the RBC membrane leading to increased extracellular potassium and free hemoglobin. Thus, the shelf life of irradiated RBCs is shortened to a maximum of 28 days from 42 days maximum shelf life. Neonates are especially vulnerable to the side effects of irradiated RBCs and the risk of hyperkalemia, especially if given in large volumes.

Washing
Washing involves RBCs being washed with 1 to 2 L of normal saline (0.9%) to remove 99% of the plasma proteins and additives and the washed RBCs are then resuspended in normal saline to a final hematocrit of 70% to 80%. The primary indications for washing are recurrent, severe allergic transfusion reactions to unwashed products, or absolute immunoglobulin A deficiency with a history of anaphylactoid/anaphylactic reaction or to reduce additives like mannitol or glycerol. It is to be noted, however, that washed RBCs have a reduced shelf life and must be transfused within 24 hours when

stored at 1 to 6°C. Also, washing is not a replacement for leukoreduction and can be performed only on cellular blood products.

Freezing and de-glycerolization

In rare cases, such as need for long-term storage of autologous RBC units or rare donor units with unusual antigenic phenotype, RBC units can be frozen. RBCs can be frozen in glycerol, a cryoprotectant for long-term storage, for up to 10 years. After thaw, glycerol must be removed before transfusion and RBCs are resuspended in 0.9% normal saline after washing with serially lower concentrations of sodium chloride. However, deglycerolized RBCs have a reduced shelf life at 1 to 6°C and must be transfused within 24 hours if prepared in an open system.

Pathogen reduction

Although RBCs are the most commonly transfused blood product; unlike platelets and plasma, a pathogen reduction (PR) RBC product is less commonly available and therefore less commonly used. PR products reduce the risk of transfusion-transmitted infection and are considered equivalent to irradiation to prevent TA-GVHD. PR RBC products are currently under investigation in ongoing trials in adults (https://clinicaltrials.gov/ct2/show/NCT03329404). A recent single-center study using pathogen-reduced RBC suspension derived from the whole blood and treated with riboflavin and UV light (RF + UV) showed clinical safety and efficacy in children with oncological and hematological diseases with comparable posttransfusion hematocrit and hemoglobin and no worsening in transfusion reactions with PR versus irradiated RBC suspension.[15]

PLATELET TRANSFUSIONS
Physiology

Thrombocytopenia is present in nearly all children with oncologic diagnoses at some point during their disease course as a result of bone marrow infiltration, chemotherapy, or associated illness, such as sepsis or disseminated intravascular coagulopathy. Children also may have qualitative platelet defects due to renal failure or antiplatelet therapy. Platelet transfusions are prescribed to prevent or treat bleeding (referred to as *prophylactic* or *therapeutic* transfusions, respectively). Although the exact epidemiology of platelet transfusions in all children with oncologic diagnoses is unknown, in a recent international study, in critically ill children with an underlying oncologic diagnosis, 71% of the platelet transfusions were given prophylactically.[16]

Similar to other blood products, the receipt of platelet transfusions is associated with significant morbidity. In a randomized control trial of platelet transfusion thresholds in neonates, those receiving platelet transfusions at a liberal threshold (therefore receiving more platelet transfusions) had a significantly increased rate of death and major bleeding at 28 days post randomization.[17] In an observational study of critically ill children (nearly half of whom had an underlying oncologic diagnosis), each additional dose of platelets (10 mL/kg) was independently associated with a 2% increase in mortality.[16] No studies have been specifically performed in pediatric oncology patients.

Indications

Several groups have developed evidence-based recommendations for platelet transfusions in pediatric oncology patients. The International Collaboration for Transfusion Medicine (ICTMG) recently published guidelines for adults and children with hypoproliferative thrombocytopenia due to primary bone marrow dyscrasias, infiltrative disorders, cytoreductive therapy, or hematopoietic stem cell transplantation.[18] Similar recommendations have been published by the American Society of Clinical Oncology (ASCO).[19,20] Both groups endorse the use of prophylactic platelet transfusion over a therapeutic-only approach in pediatric oncology patients. They base this recommendation on results from the TOPPS (Trial of Prophylactic Platelets) study in which there was a higher rate of bleeding in patients randomized to the therapeutic-only platelet transfusion arm.[21] Corroborating this evidence, a subanalysis of pediatric patients within the Platelet Dose Optimization (PLADO) study demonstrated increased rates of bleeding in children compared with their adult counterparts.[22]

Both the ICTMG and ASCO advocate for a prophylactic platelet transfusion threshold of 10×10^9/L. This recommendation is largely based on 2 adult studies that randomized patients with leukemia to thresholds of either 10 or 20×10^9/L and found no difference in morbidity or mortality between the 2 groups.[23,24] Recommendations for higher thresholds in specific clinical cases, such as veno-occlusive disease or disseminated intravascular coagulation, have less supporting evidence. Children undergoing hematopoietic stem cell transplantation for sickle cell disease are at high risk of intracranial hemorrhage and should have platelet counts of at least 50×10^9/L in the immediate posttransplant period.[25,26] However, little evidence exists to direct platelet transfusion therapy in pediatric oncology patients with clinically relevant bleeding, fever, hyperleukocytosis, infection, or receiving anticoagulation. Both groups suggest higher thresholds, but, without evidence, no definite platelet count is advocated. Furthermore, pediatric oncology patients frequently undergo procedures. However, few studies have been conducted to direct transfusion management in thrombocytopenic children undergoing bone marrow biopsy, lumbar puncture, central line placement, or surgery. Both surveys of pediatric oncologists[27] and observational data[28,29] to determine the ideal platelet count to prevent traumatic lumbar puncture are conflicting. Systematic reviews on platelet transfusions before central line placement[30] and surgical procedures[31] in thrombocytopenic patients show unclear benefit.

Dosing

Current dosing recommendations are 10 to 15 mL/kg of ideal body weight.[32] Transfusing pediatric oncology patients at the high end of this range may result in longer intervals between transfusions and higher incremental platelet count increases following transfusions.[22] In critically ill children with an underlying oncologic diagnosis, there is an independent association between an underlying oncologic diagnosis and a poor platelet increment response to platelet transfusion.[16]

Product-Specific Considerations

Leukoreduction, irradiation, and washing
Platelets can also undergo leukoreduction with the same benefits as indicated previously for RBCs and gamma irradiation to reduce the risk of TA-GVHD in susceptible populations with the same dose as RBCs. However, the expiration date of irradiated platelets is unchanged. Platelets can be suspended in platelet additive solution (PAS) (one-third original plasma content as compared with regular platelet concentrates). Removal of plasma from platelet products by storage in PAS or washing also decreases the incidence of febrile nonhemolytic transfusion reactions as well as helps prevent severe, recurrent allergic transfusion reactions.

Pathogen reduction
Psoralen compound (amotosalen) intercalates into nucleic acid and is crosslinked on exposure to UVA light. In general, it leads to significant PR for most organisms

and T-cells. PR products reduce the risk of transfusion-transmitted infections and transfusion-associated GVHD as PR products are irradiation equivalent. Although there is a clinically significant reduction in posttransfusion platelet count in patients treated with PR platelets, no significant differences in bleeding, transfusion reactions, or death were noticed when compared with non-PR platelets.[33] There is no pathogen inactivation process that has been shown to eliminate all pathogens. Certain nonenveloped viruses (eg, HAV, HEV, B19, and poliovirus) and *Bacillus cereus* spores have demonstrated resistance to the PR process.

There are limited data regarding the efficacy or safety of PR platelets in pediatric patients.[34,35] Hypersensitivity to amotosalen or other psoralens has been raised as a theoretic concern. For neonatal patients having received PR blood products and then being treated with phototherapy devices for hyperbilirubinemia, there is potential for erythema from interaction between UV light and amotosalen.[36] A recent study focused on platelet utilization and safety in a tertiary care hospital that transitioned from conventional to PR platelets showed a small, but statistically significant, increase in overall transfusions after PR platelet transfusion in pediatric patients, but not in neonates. In addition, transfusion reactions were similar for both products in all age groups as well as no rashes were reported in neonates receiving phototherapy and PR platelets.[35]

ABO matching

Platelets express ABO blood group antigens[37] and correspondingly the plasma found in platelet products may contain antibodies against A or B antigens, depending on the ABO type of the donor that may be reactive with the recipient's antigens. The benefit of ABO matching for platelet transfusions is controversial and no guidelines exist.[38–40]

PLASMA TRANSFUSIONS
Physiology

In addition to many other molecules, such as albumin, immunoglobulins, and up to 5×10^6 donor white blood cells, plasma contains coagulation factors. Generally, plasma is transfused to correct multiple coagulation factor deficiencies in patients with active bleeding (*therapeutic* transfusions) or to prevent bleeding before invasive procedures (*prophylactic* transfusions). Current guidelines suggest transfusing plasma only when the international normalized ratio (INR), the prothrombin time or the activated partial thromboplastin time (aPTT) is more than 1.5 times normal.[41,42] However, as the INR of a plasma unit is 1.1 (interquartile range, 0.9–1.3),[43] plasma transfusions dilute the patient's coagulation factors and, hence, very seldom correct abnormal coagulation tests. In critically ill children, the potential clinical benefit of plasma transfusions seems minimal when the INR is <2.5 or the aPTT is <60.[44]

On the other hand, plasma transfusions have been associated with worse outcome in numerous observational studies. In critically ill children, plasma transfusions are independently associated with increased risk of respiratory failure, multiple organ failure, nosocomial infections, and prolonged pediatric intensive care unit length of stay.[45,46] In children after liver transplantation, plasma transfusions also were associated with worse clinical outcome.[47] Although some critically ill children with underlying oncologic diagnoses were included in the large observational study,[44] no data specifically address pediatric oncology patients.

As asparaginase decreases the production of antithrombin 3 (AT3) and fibrinogen, some clinicians use prophylactic plasma transfusions in the hope of keeping these levels within the normal range. However, observational studies have shown that plasma transfusions fail to correct AT3 and fibrinogen levels in these patients[48,49] or in other situations with low AT3 levels, such as after liver transplantation.[50] Furthermore, there is no evidence that prophylactic plasma transfusions improve clinical outcome in patients receiving asparaginase.[51]

Plasma transfusions are also sometimes given to patients at risk of hepatic veno-occlusive disease (VOD), either prophylactically to prevent VOD[52] or in combination with defibrotide to treat severe VOD.[53] However, to our knowledge, there is no evidence that plasma transfusions improve the clinical outcome in these patients.

Indications

Across a range of indications, a meta-analysis of 80 randomized controlled trials demonstrated the lack of benefit for prophylactic plasma transfusion.[54] Considering that plasma transfusions have been shown to be independently associated with worse clinical outcome,[44–46] there is no evidence to support transfusing plasma solely to prevent bleeding. There are no data specifically addressing oncologic patients.

In massively bleeding patients, observational data suggest that a higher ratio of plasma (and platelets) to RBCs is associated with improved survival.[55] However, a large randomized controlled trial in adults requiring massive transfusion did not find that a plasma-platelet-RBC ratio greater than 1:1:2 improved survival.[56] In non–life-threatening bleeding, despite the lack of randomized controlled trials, it seems reasonable to transfuse plasma to patients with clinically significant bleeding and INR greater than 2.5, given that plasma transfusions fail to correct INR less than 2.5[43] and are independently associated with worse clinical outcome.[44–46]

Dosing

In a large observational study, the median dose of plasma was 11 mL/kg (interquartile range, 9.7–15.1).[43] A small randomized controlled trial in critically ill adults showed that a higher dose (20 mL/kg) was not superior to a standard dose (12 mL/kg).[57]

Product-Specific Considerations

Pathogen reduction
Pooled plasma (>1000 donors) from a single ABO group may be solvent detergent-treated to inactivate enveloped viruses and then sterile filtered to remove parasites and bacteria and tested for hepatitis E and parvovirus B19. There is a slight but clinically nonsignificant reduction in most coagulation factors with solvent detergent treatment, except protein S and alpha-2-antiplasmin, which are destroyed. Use of solvent detergent plasma compared with fresh frozen plasma/frozen plasma-24 hour has been associated with improved survival in critically ill pediatric patients.[58]

GRANULOCYTE TRANSFUSIONS

Pediatric oncology patients may develop severe and prolonged neutropenia. Although no clear guidelines or studies confirming effectiveness exist, granulocyte transfusions may be considered in children with an absolute neutrophil count less than 500/μL or known neutrophil dysfunction AND an invasive clinical infection with proven inadequate response to antimicrobial therapy. It is only supposed to be a transient bridging support and not a life-prolonging measure. Thus, granulocyte transfusions are recommended only in situations in which there is a reasonable chance of marrow recovery.[59] Adverse reactions are common and may include fever, hypotension, and respiratory insufficiency.[60] A systematic review published in 2016, which included mostly adult subjects, failed to find any benefit on the survival rate or the number of people who recover from an infection.[61]

Table 1
Overview of indications and dosing for blood products in pediatric oncology patients

Blood Product	Indications	Dosing	Processing Considerations
RBC	Hemoglobin <7–8 g/dL	10–15 mL/kg	Leukoreduction Irradiation Washing
Platelets	Platelet count <10 × 10^9/L OR clinically significant bleeding	10–15 mL/kg	Leukoreduction Irradiation (or consider pathogen reduction) Washing Consider ABO matching Volume reduction
Plasma	INR >2.5 AND clinically significant bleeding	10 mL/kg	Pathogen reduction Volume reduction (lower dosing)

Abbreviations: INR, international normalized ratio; RBC, red blood cell.

SUMMARY

Pediatric oncology patients will likely require numerous transfusions of blood products during the course of their treatment (**Table 1**). Although strong evidence-based guidelines for this patient population do not exist, given the morbidities associated with the receipt of blood products, practitioners should attempt to use restrictive transfusion strategies.

REFERENCES

1. Weiskopf RB, Viele MK, Feiner J, et al. Human cardiovascular and metabolic response to acute, severe isovolemic anemia. JAMA 1998;279(3):217–21.
2. Carson JL, Noveck H, Berlin JA, et al. Mortality and morbidity in patients with very low postoperative Hb levels who decline blood transfusion. Transfusion 2002; 42(7):812–8.
3. Vincent JL, Baron JF, Reinhart K, et al. Anemia and blood transfusion in critically ill patients. JAMA 2002;288(12):1499–507.
4. Kneyber MC, Hersi MI, Twisk JW, et al. Red blood cell transfusion in critically ill children is independently associated with increased mortality. Intensive Care Med 2007;33(8):1414–22.
5. Bateman ST, Lacroix J, Boven K, et al. Anemia, blood loss, and blood transfusions in North American children in the intensive care unit. Am J Respir Crit Care Med 2008;178(1):26–33.
6. New HV, Grant-Casey J, Lowe D, et al. Red blood cell transfusion practice in children: current status and areas for improvement? A study of the use of red blood cell transfusions in children and infants. Transfusion 2014;54(1):119–27.
7. Steiner ME, Zantek ND, Stanworth SJ, et al. Recommendations on RBC transfusion support in children with hematologic and oncologic diagnoses from the pediatric critical care transfusion and anemia expertise initiative. Pediatr Crit Care Med 2018;19(9S Suppl 1):S149–56.
8. Lightdale JR, Randolph AG, Tran CM, et al. Impact of a conservative red blood cell transfusion strategy in children undergoing hematopoietic stem cell transplantation. Biol Blood Marrow Transplant 2012;18(5):813–7.

9. International Society of Blood Transfusion. Single unit transfusion. Available at: http://www.isbtweb.org/working-parties/clinical-transfusion/6-single-unit-transfusion/. Accessed November 28, 2018.

10. Bowman Z, Cumpston A, Craig M, et al. Single unit red blood cell transfusion is a safe and effective alternative to double unit transfusion in hematologic malignancies. Blood 2016;128(22):383–8.

11. AABB. Circular of information for the use of human blood and blood components 2017. Available at: https://marketplace.aabb.org/ebusiness/Default.aspx?TabID=251&productId=13452514.

12. King KE, Shirey RS, Thoman SK, et al. Universal leukoreduction decreases the incidence of febrile nonhemolytic transfusion reactions to RBCs. Transfusion 2004;44(1):25–9.

13. Paglino JC, Pomper GJ, Fisch GS, et al. Reduction of febrile but not allergic reactions to RBCs and platelets after conversion to universal prestorage leukoreduction. Transfusion 2004;44(1):16–24.

14. Ruhl H, Bein G, Sachs UJ. Transfusion-associated graft-versus-host disease. Transfus Med Rev 2009;23(1):62–71.

15. Trakhtman P, Kumukova I, Starostin N, et al. The pathogen-reduced red blood cell suspension: single centre study of clinical safety and efficacy in children with oncological and haematological diseases. Vox Sang 2019;114(3):223–31.

16. Nellis ME, Karam O, Mauer E, et al. Platelet transfusion practices in critically ill children. Crit Care Med 2018;46(8):1309–17.

17. Curley A, Stanworth SJ, Willoughby K, et al. Randomized trial of platelet-transfusion thresholds in neonates. N Engl J Med 2019;380(3):242–51.

18. Nahirniak S, Slichter SJ, Tanael S, et al. Guidance on platelet transfusion for patients with hypoproliferative thrombocytopenia. Transfus Med Rev 2015;29(1):3–13.

19. Schiffer CA, Anderson KC, Bennett CL, et al. Platelet transfusion for patients with cancer: clinical practice guidelines of the American Society of Clinical Oncology. J Clin Oncol 2001;19(5):1519–38.

20. Schiffer CA, Bohlke K, Delaney M, et al. Platelet transfusion for patients with cancer: American Society of Clinical Oncology clinical practice guideline update. J Clin Oncol 2018;36(3):283–99.

21. Stanworth SJ, Estcourt LJ, Powter G, et al. A no-prophylaxis platelet-transfusion strategy for hematologic cancers. N Engl J Med 2013;368(19):1771–80.

22. Josephson CD, Granger S, Assmann SF, et al. Bleeding risks are higher in children versus adults given prophylactic platelet transfusions for treatment-induced hypoproliferative thrombocytopenia. Blood 2012;120(4):748–60.

23. Heckman KD, Weiner GJ, Davis CS, et al. Randomized study of prophylactic platelet transfusion threshold during induction therapy for adult acute leukemia: 10,000/microL versus 20,000/microL. J Clin Oncol 1997;15(3):1143–9.

24. Rebulla P, Finazzi G, Marangoni F, et al. The threshold for prophylactic platelet transfusions in adults with acute myeloid leukemia. Gruppo Italiano Malattie Ematologiche Maligne dell'Adulto. N Engl J Med 1997;337(26):1870–5.

25. Bernaudin F, Socie G, Kuentz M, et al. Long-term results of related myeloablative stem-cell transplantation to cure sickle cell disease. Blood 2007;110(7):2749–56.

26. McPherson ME, Anderson AR, Haight AE, et al. Transfusion management of sickle cell patients during bone marrow transplantation with matched sibling donor. Transfusion 2009;49(9):1977–86.

27. Wong EC, Perez-Albuerne E, Moscow JA, et al. Transfusion management strategies: a survey of practicing pediatric hematology/oncology specialists. Pediatr Blood Cancer 2005;44(2):119–27.

28. Howard SC, Gajjar A, Ribeiro RC, et al. Safety of lumbar puncture for children with acute lymphoblastic leukemia and thrombocytopenia. JAMA 2000;284(17):2222–4.

29. Howard SC, Gajjar AJ, Cheng C, et al. Risk factors for traumatic and bloody lumbar puncture in children with acute lymphoblastic leukemia. JAMA 2002;288(16): 2001–7.

30. van de Weerdt EK, Biemond BJ, Baake B, et al. Central venous catheter placement in coagulopathic patients: risk factors and incidence of bleeding complications. Transfusion 2017;57(10):2512–25.

31. Estcourt LJ, Malouf R, Doree C, et al. Prophylactic platelet transfusions prior to surgery for people with a low platelet count. Cochrane Database Syst Rev 2018;(9):CD012779.

32. Josephson CD, Sloan SR. Pediatric transfusion medicine. In: Hoffman R, Benz EJ, Silberstein LE, editors. Hematology: basic principles and practice. 6th edition. Philadelphia: Elsevier; 2013. p. 1765–71.

33. Rebulla P, Vaglio S, Beccaria F, et al. Clinical effectiveness of platelets in additive solution treated with two commercial pathogen-reduction technologies. Transfusion 2017;57(5):1171–83.

34. Jacquot C, Delaney M. Pathogen-inactivated blood products for pediatric patients: blood safety, patient safety, or both? Transfusion 2018;58(9):2095–101.

35. Schulz WL, McPadden J, Gehrie EA, et al. Blood utilization and transfusion reactions in pediatric patients transfused with conventional or pathogen reduced platelets. J Pediatr 2019. https://doi.org/10.1016/j.jpeds.2019.01.046.

36. Corporation C. INTERCEPT® Blood System for Platelets–Large Volume (LV) Processing Set. [Package Insert]. 2018; SPC 00698-AW, V2.0:Package insert. Available at: https://www.intercept-usa.com/warnings-and-contraindications. Accessed October 28, 2018.

37. Cooling LL, Kelly K, Barton J, et al. Determinants of ABH expression on human blood platelets. Blood 2005;105(8):3356–64.

38. Solves P, Carpio N, Balaguer A, et al. Transfusion of ABO non-identical platelets does not influence the clinical outcome of patients undergoing autologous haematopoietic stem cell transplantation. Blood Transfus 2015;13(3):411–6.

39. Shehata N, Tinmouth A, Naglie G, et al. ABO-identical versus nonidentical platelet transfusion: a systematic review. Transfusion 2009;49(11):2442–53.

40. Nellis ME, Goel R, Karam O, et al. Effects of ABO matching of platelet transfusions in critically ill children. Pediatr Crit Care Med 2019;20(2):e61–9.

41. O'Shaughnessy DF, Atterbury C, Bolton Maggs P, et al. Guidelines for the use of fresh-frozen plasma, cryoprecipitate and cryosupernatant. Br J Haematol 2004; 126(1):11–28.

42. Liumbruno G, Bennardello F, Lattanzio A, et al. Recommendations for the transfusion of plasma and platelets. Blood Transfus 2009;7(2):132–50.

43. Holland LL, Foster TM, Marlar RA, et al. Fresh frozen plasma is ineffective for correcting minimally elevated international normalized ratios. Transfusion 2005; 45(7):1234–5.

44. Karam O, Demaret P, Shefler A, et al. Indications and effects of plasma transfusions in critically ill children. Am J Respir Crit Care Med 2015;191(12):1395–402.

45. Church GD, Matthay MA, Liu K, et al. Blood product transfusions and clinical outcomes in pediatric patients with acute lung injury. Pediatr Crit Care Med 2009; 10(3):297–302.

46. Karam O, Lacroix J, Robitaille N, et al. Association between plasma transfusions and clinical outcome in critically ill children: a prospective observational study. Vox Sang 2013;104(4):342–9.
47. Nacoti M, Cazzaniga S, Lorusso F, et al. The impact of perioperative transfusion of blood products on survival after pediatric liver transplantation. Pediatr Transplant 2012;16(4):357–66.
48. Halton JM, Mitchell LG, Vegh P, et al. Fresh frozen plasma has no beneficial effect on the hemostatic system in children receiving L-asparaginase. Am J Hematol 1994;47(3):157–61.
49. Nowak-Gottl U, Rath B, Binder M, et al. Inefficacy of fresh frozen plasma in the treatment of L-asparaginase-induced coagulation factor deficiencies during ALL induction therapy. Haematologica 1995;80(5):451–3.
50. Arni D, Wildhaber BE, McLin V, et al. Effects of plasma transfusions on antithrombin levels after paediatric liver transplantation. Vox Sang 2018. [Epub ahead of print].
51. Abbott LS, Deevska M, Fernandez CV, et al. The impact of prophylactic fresh-frozen plasma and cryoprecipitate on the incidence of central nervous system thrombosis and hemorrhage in children with acute lymphoblastic leukemia receiving asparaginase. Blood 2009;114(25):5146–51.
52. Matsumoto M, Kawa K, Uemura M, et al. Prophylactic fresh frozen plasma may prevent development of hepatic VOD after stem cell transplantation via ADAMTS13-mediated restoration of von Willebrand factor plasma levels. Bone Marrow Transplant 2007;40(3):251–9.
53. Richardson PG, Soiffer RJ, Antin JH, et al. Defibrotide for the treatment of severe hepatic veno-occlusive disease and multiorgan failure after stem cell transplantation: a multicenter, randomized, dose-finding trial. Biol Blood Marrow Transplant 2010;16(7):1005–17.
54. Yang L, Stanworth S, Hopewell S, et al. Is fresh-frozen plasma clinically effective? An update of a systematic review of randomized controlled trials. Transfusion 2012;52(8):1673–86 [quiz: 1673].
55. Holcomb JB, Wade CE, Michalek JE, et al. Increased plasma and platelet to red blood cell ratios improves outcome in 466 massively transfused civilian trauma patients. Ann Surg 2008;248(3):447–58.
56. Holcomb JB, Tilley BC, Baraniuk S, et al. Transfusion of plasma, platelets, and red blood cells in a 1:1:1 vs a 1:1:2 ratio and mortality in patients with severe trauma: the PROPPR randomized clinical trial. JAMA 2015;313(5):471–82.
57. Tinmouth A, Chatelain E, Fergusson D, et al. A randomized controlled trial of high and standard dose frozen plasma transfusions in critically ill patients. Transfusion 2008;48S:26A–7A.
58. Camazine MN, Karam O, Colvin R, et al. Outcomes related to the use of frozen plasma or pooled solvent/detergent-treated plasma in critically ill children. Pediatr Crit Care Med 2017;18(5):e215–23.
59. Marfin AA, Price TH. Granulocyte transfusion therapy. J Intensive Care Med 2015; 30(2):79–88.
60. Grigull L, Pulver N, Goudeva L, et al. G-CSF mobilised granulocyte transfusions in 32 paediatric patients with neutropenic sepsis. Support Care Cancer 2006;14(9): 910–6.
61. Estcourt LJ, Stanworth SJ, Hopewell S, et al. Granulocyte transfusions for treating infections in people with neutropenia or neutrophil dysfunction. Cochrane Database Syst Rev 2016;(4):CD005339.

UNITED STATES POSTAL SERVICE ® Statement of Ownership, Management, and Circulation (All Periodicals Publications Except Requester Publications)

1. Publication Title	2. Publication Number	3. Filing Date
HEMATOLOGY/ONCOLOGY CLINICS OF NORTH AMERICA	002 – 473	9/18/2019

4. Issue Frequency	5. Number of Issues Published Annually	6. Annual Subscription Price
FEB, APR, JUN, AUG, OCT, DEC	6	$430.00

7. Complete Mailing Address of Known Office of Publication (Not printer) (Street, city, county, state, and ZIP+4®)

ELSEVIER INC.
230 Park Avenue, Suite 800
New York, NY 10169

Contact Person
STEPHEN R. BUSHING

Telephone (Include area code)
215-239-3688

8. Complete Mailing Address of Headquarters or General Business Office of Publisher (Not printer)

ELSEVIER INC.
230 Park Avenue, Suite 800
New York, NY 10169

9. Full Names and Complete Mailing Addresses of Publisher, Editor, and Managing Editor (Do not leave blank)

Publisher (Name and complete mailing address)

TAYLOR BALL, ELSEVIER INC.
1600 JOHN F KENNEDY BLVD. SUITE 1800
PHILADELPHIA, PA 19103-2899

Editor (Name and complete mailing address)

STACY EASTMAN, ELSEVIER INC.
1600 JOHN F KENNEDY BLVD. SUITE 1800
PHILADELPHIA, PA 19103-2899

Managing Editor (Name and complete mailing address)

PATRICK MANLEY, ELSEVIER INC.
1600 JOHN F KENNEDY BLVD. SUITE 1800
PHILADELPHIA, PA 19103-2899

10. Owner (Do not leave blank. If the publication is owned by a corporation, give the name and address of the corporation immediately followed by the names and addresses of all stockholders owning or holding 1 percent or more of the total amount of stock. If not owned by a corporation, give the names and addresses of the individual owners. If owned by a partnership or other unincorporated firm, give its name and address as well as those of each individual owner. If the publication is published by a nonprofit organization, give its name and address.)

Full Name	Complete Mailing Address
WHOLLY OWNED SUBSIDIARY OF REED/ELSEVIER, US HOLDINGS	1600 JOHN F KENNEDY BLVD. SUITE 1800 PHILADELPHIA, PA 19103-2899

11. Known Bondholders, Mortgagees, and Other Security Holders Owning or Holding 1 Percent or More of Total Amount of Bonds, Mortgages, or Other Securities. If none, check box ► ☐ None

Full Name	Complete Mailing Address
N/A	

12. Tax Status (For completion by nonprofit organizations authorized to mail at nonprofit rates) (Check one)
The purpose, function, and nonprofit status of this organization and the exempt status for federal income tax purposes:
☒ Has Not Changed During Preceding 12 Months
☐ Has Changed During Preceding 12 Months (Publisher must submit explanation of change with this statement)

PS Form 3526, July 2014 [Page 1 of 4 (see instructions page 4)] PSN: 7530-01-000-9931 PRIVACY NOTICE: See our privacy policy on www.usps.com.

13. Publication Title	14. Issue Date for Circulation Data Below
HEMATOLOGY/ONCOLOGY CLINICS OF NORTH AMERICA	JUNE 2019

15. Extent and Nature of Circulation			Average No. Copies Each Issue During Preceding 12 Months	No. Copies of Single Issue Published Nearest to Filing Date
a. Total Number of Copies (Net press run)			177	173
b. Paid Circulation (By Mail and Outside the Mail)	(1)	Mailed Outside-County Paid Subscriptions Stated on PS Form 3541 (Include paid distribution above nominal rate, advertiser's proof copies, and exchange copies)	55	64
	(2)	Mailed In-County Paid Subscriptions Stated on PS Form 3541 (Include paid distribution above nominal rate, advertiser's proof copies, and exchange copies)	0	0
	(3)	Paid Distribution Outside the Mails Including Sales Through Dealers and Carriers, Street Vendors, Counter Sales, and Other Paid Distribution Outside USPS®	40	53
	(4)	Paid Distribution by Other Classes of Mail Through the USPS (e.g., First-Class Mail®)	0	0
c. Total Paid Distribution (Sum of 15b (1), (2), (3), and (4))			95	117
d. Free or Nominal Rate Distribution (By Mail and Outside the Mail)	(1)	Free or Nominal Rate Outside-County Copies included on PS Form 3541	70	42
	(2)	Free or Nominal Rate In-County Copies Included on PS Form 3541	0	0
	(3)	Free or Nominal Rate Copies Mailed at Other Classes Through the USPS (e.g., First-Class Mail)	0	0
	(4)	Free or Nominal Rate Distribution Outside the Mail (Carriers or other means)	0	0
e. Total Free or Nominal Rate Distribution (Sum of 15d (1), (2), (3) and (4))			70	42
f. Total Distribution (Sum of 15c and 15e)			165	159
g. Copies not Distributed (See Instructions to Publishers #4 (page 83))			12	14
h. Total (Sum of 15f and g)			177	173
i. Percent Paid (15c divided by 15f times 100)			57.58%	73.58%

* If you are claiming electronic copies, go to line 16 on page 3. If you are not claiming electronic copies, skip to line 17 on page 3.

16. Electronic Copy Circulation	Average No. Copies Each Issue During Preceding 12 Months	No. Copies of Single Issue Published Nearest to Filing Date
a. Paid Electronic Copies ►		
b. Total Paid Print Copies (Line 15c) + Paid Electronic Copies (Line 16a) ►		
c. Total Print Distribution (Line 15f) + Paid Electronic Copies (Line 16a) ►		
d. Percent Paid (Both Print & Electronic Copies) (16b divided by 16c × 100) ►		

☒ I certify that 50% of all my distributed copies (electronic and print) are paid above a nominal price.

17. Publication of Statement of Ownership
☒ If the publication is a general publication, publication of this statement is required. Will be printed ☐ Publication not required.
in the OCTOBER 2019 issue of this publication.

18. Signature and Title of Editor, Publisher, Business Manager, or Owner

STEPHEN R. BUSHING - INVENTORY DISTRIBUTION CONTROL MANAGER

Stephen R. Bushing Date 9/18/2019

I certify that all information furnished on this form is true and complete. I understand that anyone who furnishes false or misleading information on this form or who omits material or information requested on the form may be subject to criminal sanctions (including fines and imprisonment) and/or civil sanctions (including civil penalties).

PS Form 3526, July 2014 (Page 3 of 4) PRIVACY NOTICE: See our privacy policy on www.usps.com.

Printed and bound by CPI Group (UK) Ltd, Croydon, CR0 4YY

03/10/2024

01040404-0016